Drinking-Water and Ice Supplies

Also from Westphalia Press
westphaliapress.org

Drinking-Water and Ice Supplies

and Their Relations to Health and Disease: Filtration in the 1900s

by
T. Mitchell Prudden, MD

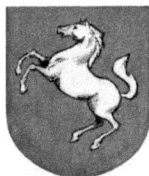

WESTPHALIA PRESS
An Imprint of Policy Studies Organization

Westphalia Press
An imprint of Policy Studies Organization
1527 New Hampshire Ave., NW
Washington, D.C. 20036
info@ipsonet.org

ISBN-13: 978-1-63391-532-9
ISBN-10: 1-63391-532-8

Cover design by Jeffrey Barnes:
jbarnesbook.design

Daniel Gutierrez-Sandoval, Executive Director
PSO and Westphalia Press

Updated material and comments on this edition
can be found at the Westphalia Press website:
www.westphaliapress.org

DRINKING-WATER AND ICE SUPPLIES

AND THEIR

RELATIONS TO HEALTH AND DISEASE

BY

T. MITCHELL PRUDDEN, M.D.

AUTHOR OF "THE STORY OF THE BACTERIA," "DUST AND ITS DANGERS," ETC.

SECOND EDITION

G. P. PUTNAM'S SONS

NEW YORK   LONDON
27 WEST TWENTY-THIRD ST. 24 BEDFORD ST., STRAND
The Knickerbocker Press
1901

The Knickerbocker Press, New York

PREFACE.

THIS little book has been written with the purpose of informing the householder how wholesome water may be obtained both in town and country. This end is sought not by laying down a series of axioms and rules, but rather by calling the reader's attention to some more or less interesting facts about water and water supplies, in the hope of helping him on these to base an independent judgment applicable to his own particular case. Some of the new bacterial lore is brought into prominence, because a good deal of the current distrust of good water sources arises from false notions as to the relationships of the water-bacteria to disease. On the other hand, it is believed that much serious illness may be spared by a knowledge of such facts as are here laid down about the real dangers which lurk in water made impure by inattention to simple sanitary laws.

T. M. P.

CONTENTS

ILLUSTRATIONS

DRINKING-WATER AND ICE SUPPLIES

AND THEIR

RELATIONS TO HEALTH AND DISEASE.

CHAPTER I.

PLANS AND PURPOSES.

I T is neither the purpose nor the hope of the writer of this little book to say any thing especially new or any thing startling about water. Nor does he plan to set in array the many varied properties which make it at once one of the most useful and beautiful and indispensable to life, of all the forms of created things. He wishes only to ask his reader to consider with him, in the light of some of the new and marvellous discoveries of modern science, sundry relationships which water bears to civilized life, and some of the ways in which we are enabled to supply ourselves with it, both for cleanliness and nourishment, in pure and wholesome form.

There is a legend of a sprite in the Thuringian forest, whom the people suspected of hostile intent, and in order to assure them of his harmlessness and good feeling, he was wont, when he met them, to take off his skull and show them that it was hollow. While deprecating a too literal analogy between the anatomical characteristics of this being and himself, the writer would still wish as clearly to absolve himself from the charge of sheer wantonness and to expose his intent in writing for unscientific people a book which contains, among other things, a few very disquieting revelations about some people's drinking-water.

There are a good many fancies and beliefs about drinking-water, which are founded in ignorance, perpetuated by indifference, and culminate in serious physical disorders. These the writer wishes to expose and combat.

There have been many new and important revelations within the past few years about the relations of good water to good health, and of bad water to varying degrees of bad health. These, with what clearness he can master, the writer purposes to set forth.

There are a good many simple suggestions which from our new vantage-ground can be made to the householder, both in town and country, as to what good water is, how he may secure it for his domestic use, and how he may judge of the probabilities of danger in a suspected supply. To make these suggestions is the most practical purpose of this little book.

Finally, the writer would call the attention of those who object to being reminded of their accustomed sanitary misdeeds, to the fact that the medical science of to-day is raising its standard of advance with this conviction that widespread prevention, when it is possible, is better than cure. A large measure of prevention is possible in many serious diseases, which have been always and abundantly with us, because we have not known until now just what caused them and how to curtail their spread.

If anybody thinks life is not worth living because he is advised to walk on one side of a street to avoid falling bricks on the other, he is one, it may be frankly said, for whom this book is not written.   It is for those who, taking the world as it is, are concerned to make it as much better as they can ; for those who can see, without elaborate explanation, that sanitary savagery does not well accord with that cleanly living which is a distinguishing mark of civilization ; for those who are not too indolent or engaged to look fairly at the reasons which have given rise to the general demand, so frequent to-day, for clean food, clean water, clean air, clean surroundings, and the physical and mental vigor which these conditions foster.

The various departments of science are so closely interlinked that achievements in each throw light upon the problems of the others, often in very unexpected ways.   And so if the reader finds that now and then we have left the water-ways and are wandering inland ; if we seem to lose from sight for a moment the evident practical ends of our special study, to spy out some secrets of the solid earth ; if now and then we step aside for a little, to watch curiously the student in his laboratory, as he probes, and peers, and ponders, we should not forget that so only can we fit ourselves to form independent judgments,—so only be masters of our subject. and not mere Gradgrinds of the hour.

CHAPTER II

GLIMPSES OF A WORLD'S WORKSHOP.

ASTRONOMERS and physicists tell us that the material which forms our world was once poised in space as a vast, fiery, cloud-like mass of nebulous vapor. They tell us that, little by little as the ages rolled away, this "fire-mist," under the influence of well-known physical laws, grew denser and denser, until it was largely concentrated into the solid groundwork of a new planet. This new planet, red-hot from Nature's workshop in space, slowly cooled upon the outside, and, after much turmoil and with titanic throes which tore and scarred and seamed the new-formed crust, at length gave up for the most part its struggle and strife, and entered upon an orderly career, as a staid, solid, reliable world.

There seems, however, to have been left

over, after the foundations were laid, a certain amount of matter, mostly in the form of gases and fluids, which has assumed, as the world's history has gone on developing, a most important, if not a dominant, rôle.

When the chemists pull this residual world-matter to pieces, they find that it is largely made up of a few simple elementary substances, which they call carbon, hydrogen, oxygen, and nitrogen,—partly free, but mostly in varying combinations with one another. One of the most abundant and widespread of these combinations is that of oxygen and hydrogen in water—now invisible as gas or steam, again taking form in clouds, or lingering most willingly as the fluid which we know so well, or growing hard and cold in ice.

Before the new old earth, self-luminous then, had cooled, the water, far diffused in space as a gas, was invisible. But when the temperature had sufficiently fallen, it began to assume the form of vapor—visible as condensing steam or clouds, had there been eyes to see it. These clouds grew denser and denser, wholly veiling the sun, no doubt, and forming a lurid canopy over the but partially cooled globe. It will be remembered that at this time there was no sea, there were no lakes, no streams— all that vast quantity of water, which we know so well to-day, hung poised over the earth, still too hot to hold it for an instant upon its surface.

Then as the earth still further cooled, there came an age of rain and storms, so fierce and wild, that we can form no adequate conception of its fury. The hot earth sent back the hissing torrents which had formed above, over and over and over again, until finally a boiling, shoreless sea had gained its watery foothold, and then, slowly, but at last, the clouds cleared away, and the earth, itself no longer shining, beheld its sun—our sun to-day.

With what further writhings and struggles the panting earth made special place for the waters upon its surface, and the dry, cool land —all rock—appeared, let the geologist tell us, if he will or can.

At any rate, the ages rolled on, and at some time or other, when or how, we do not know, under what forces, natural or Divine—which is perhaps the same thing,—we can only conjecture, a marvellous influence came upon some of these same residual elements of a world's building, and fostered in them a potency which we call life—a potency which has remained, self-renewing, intangible, and as mysterious as at its first dawn upon the new earth.

It is, after all, life and living things alone which give, for us at any rate, special significance to this great sphere, bowling on through space so monotonously from age to age. And when we come to think of it, it is only just a little thin, uneven shell outside of the solid surface of the earth—the outer layers of the soil and the surface waters—which foster and contain the consummation of our world's powers and wild experiences—living things.

Bound up so closely with those forms of matter in which life finds expression, that life cannot be conceived of as active without it, and making up so large a part of living things, that it dominates all their other elements, water is as indispensable to life, as are the forces which have made life a world's chiefest adornment and its master.

It would require the scientist's knowledge, the poet's insight, and a master's pen to portray the wonderful changes and vicissitudes of a single drop of water, as in its own form it soars in the clouds, or falls in rain, or yields itself to the thirsty earth ; to trace its transmutation into a vital factor of a living cell in animal or plant ; to show, how wooed by the rootlet in the soil to its embrace, with what silent but resistless force its atoms are torn asunder, and find themselves at length in new combination, swaying in the sunshine as a part of petal, leaf, or stem.

And so it would seem that while the great mass of the old primitive nebula has sunk to rest at last in the solid rock, or has become pent up still uncooled at the earth's centre, that poor residuum which swept over the cooling continents as water with such resistless force for so many ages, and those other elements which were called by a more exalted destiny to share in the expression of life, are still ceaselessly at work in shaping those factors which make our world more than a mere mass of inanimate matter.

It is interesting to notice that those elements which we have called residual in the world's making, the water as well as the other elements which enter into the structure of living things, are in a state of ceaseless activity, and are being used over and over again in forming and maintaining the varied kinds of life. For a period, brief as the waves' poise, they are held in the domain of life, and then comes death and disintegration. But this life-stuff is precious and not very abundant, and so again and again it falls under the spell of the life forces and shares anew in the domination of the world. In truth, that rejected elemental matter from a world's workshop has become the corner-stone to that fairer structure which we may call the living earth.

But we must not linger longer upon these heights ; these are practical times, and most people want something more definite than the vagaries of a star-gazer, who is soon jostled out of the way, if he have not things more practical to offer than far horizons and inspiring points of view.

CHAPTER III.

ALL the available water in the world—the water which is not being temporarily made use of by living things, or is not locked up in the structure of the rocks or in other chemical combinations—is either floating in the atmosphere, or flowing or lying on the earth's surface, or hidden more or less deeply within or beneath the soil.

In primitive, newly settled countries, people get water for their personal uses, as a rule, wherever they happen to find it, in lakes and streams or springs, and the presence of these water sources has, as everybody knows, been a very important factor in determining where communities shall settle and form centres of growth. But as time has gone on, men and communities have learned in a measure to

coerce nature. So it has come about that any-
where and everywhere the standard of residence may be planted at the dictates of every
possible motive, and in one way or another,
for better or worse, water, for man's personal
uses, is made to be forthcoming.

How much water on an average an individual needs in civilized life for personal and
domestic uses depends a good deal, of course,
upon his habits and occupations, as well as
upon the character of his residence. In general, it is estimated that from fifteen to twenty
gallons per day for each person is a reasonable
amount. But when to these more limited uses
of water we add the amounts needed for manufacturing purposes, for street cleaning, for
extinguishing fires, for fountains, etc., a much
larger quantity will be required. About sixty
gallons per day per person has been regarded
as sufficient, by competent authorities, for all
these various purposes.

In many towns in this country the average
supply is larger than this. In New York, for
example, it is estimated that we have, or are
soon to have at least, as much as one hundred

gallons per head. But here an enormous amount is used in manufacturing and for motive power, and an enormous amount is most wickedly allowed to run to waste.

When we try to group the varied sources of water supply for domestic and general use, we find that they may be conveniently arranged as follows : First, rain-water, collected in cisterns ; second, surface waters, such as streams, lakes, and ponds ; third, shallow wells of the ordinary form and the common springs of superficial origin ; and finally, fourth, water which comes from a considerable depth in the earth, as from very deep wells, so-called artesian wells, and deep springs. As to the qualities and peculiarities of water from these varied sources, those we will consider by and by.

The water which falls in rain may, when it comes down upon rocky surfaces, either sink in part into cracks and fissures and so sometimes goes down to great depths in the earth, or it may run directly off into streams and ponds and lakes, or stay in puddles until it evaporates.

Rain-water and such surface water as that

of lakes and streams we need not stop to consider now, but in order to understand the water which comes from subterranean regions and forms one of the most universal sources of supply, we must make a little side study of the ground in which such waters are collected and stored. We must, in other words, come back again briefly to the Mother Earth.

CHAPTER IV.

HIDDEN WATER.

WE were prematurely hurried off from our glimpses of the old world a-building by the perhaps only fancied necessity of showing some of our friends that this was not after all a treatise on elementary geology. Having thrown a sop to the demon of the practical by this glance at drinking-waters, let us slip quietly back a few hundred or thousand millions of years, more or less, and see how it fares with the old planet, which we left slowly cooling, with its few surface wrinkles jutting above the nearly universal sea, as low storm-beaten, wave-washed mountains.

In those days great tidal waves, of several hundred feet in height, swept round and round the world. No wonder that the first lands which peered above the waters were torn and eroded and ground to powder, and that great deposits of rock *débris* were laid down beneath the water to become baked and re-crystallized, perhaps over and over again. The sea was a vast caldron, too, in which chemical combinations and recombinations between one element and another of the old earth matter went on age after age, forming great beds of sedimentary rock. But finally there emerged from the turmoil some continents which came to stay and formed the backbone of our finally firm earth crust.

We do not need to linger here to watch the geologic ages as they pass, each bringing the earth nearer to its present condition. It only concerns us to know that gradually the formative changes in the solid-rock crust, for the most part, ceased, and that piled on top of the uneven rock surface of the earth—save in the comparatively few places where it still tastes the sun—are the great beds of rock-ruins, which we call stones, boulders, pebbles, gravel, sand, clay, loam, soil.

These have been formed out of the old rocks under the influence of alternating heat

2

and cold, of water and ice, and various chemical recombinations.   We usually find them in layers of varying thickness, called strata, the size of the rock fragment often varying in the different adjacent layers.   Their stratified character is largely due to the fact that they were formed when the country was covered with water.

Go into the garden and pick up a handful of dirt or sand, and look at the particles which make it up, with a magnifying-glass, and you would find, could you but read their stories, such strange experiences, such a history of rock wreckage, such records of heat and cold, of storm and lightning and pressure and chemical diablery, as would make your head swim.   You may seem almost to hear the thunder of that primeval ocean, as it rolled in upon the emerging granite cliff, and tore off this little quartz fragment.   It has since been rolled upon the beaches of unnamed seas, and swept in floods along vanished river-beds. Frozen fast in the great glaciers, it has been ground along for hundreds of miles over the old rock surfaces, scratching them as it went, until now, far from its home, a tiny glass-like particle, it has come to rest at the door with myriads of its fellows, of kindred experiences, as a part of your acre.

In the superficial layers of the soil the rock-ruin particles are variously mingled with fragments of dead vegetable and animal material and particles of organic matter of various kinds, thus making the loam or mould which is suited for the support of living plants. We thus have for the purpose of our present study to consider the earth as having, first, a rock surface, for the most part, impervious to water, save where here and there it finds its way between the strata or into caverns or fissures ; and, second, outside of this a soil surface which in contour corresponds only in a very general way with the rock surface lying at varying distances beneath.

In most regions then a more or less porous envelope spreads itself over the solid earth. This porous envelope of loam or sand or gravel is very frequently interrupted, as one follows it downward, by layers of clay impervious to water, which form more or less extensive, often bowl-like, shelves on which the water which soaks through the porous soil collects. Layers of solid rock, too, not infrequently lie interspersed with porous-soil layers, and all often slope in varying directions.

Now we are very apt to think of the soil which covers the earth as a very good material for plants to take root and grow in, and when we have considered how the plant rootlets take up food and water from the soil, we are apt to think that we have exhausted the study of its activities, and that all below the surface is dark and still and passive as the underlying rock itself.

But this is very far from being true. In the first place, the fragments or particles which make up the soil are so irregular in shape that even when closely packed they always leave spaces between them filled with air ; these air spaces are often very small when the earth particles are fine,—larger when the solid particles are larger. This air between the particles of the soil is called " ground air," and when the soil is deep there may be in the aggregate a real subterranean atmosphere of great extent. This ground air, as a whole, is not exactly the same in composition as that we breathe, because it is apt to contain more carbonic acid and less oxygen, and in cities where there are leaky gas pipes, may contain a good deal of illuminating gas.

This underground air is, however, almost as ceaselessly in motion as is that in which we move. Whenever the ground gets heated, it streams out of the myriad pores of the surface into the sunshine. When the ground cools, back through the same pores rushes the aërial air. Every wind which sweeps the surface moves the air beneath in great volumes. With every rain it is driven deeper down. The movements of this buried atmosphere are slow, because it must find its way around the myriads of soil particles which block its course. But it is of great extent and of great importance, as we shall see by and by.

But it is not with air alone that the soil pores are filled. They form the great land reservoirs of water. When the rain falls on the dry porous soil, for a time at least, a good deal of it soaks into it, displacing the air, driving it out, or sideways, or deeper down. If the rain continue, deeper and deeper trickle the drops through loam or sand or gravel, until at last they reach an impervious layer, such as rock or clay, and here may collect, if the surface be suitable, in larger or smaller sub-terranean puddles or ponds or lakes ; or if these impervious strata slope, may form broad, slowly flowing underground streams, which at last empty into some surface body of water, such as a river or a lake, at a lower level.

This subterranean water, either still or flowing, is called "ground water," so that almost everywhere we go we are not only treading upon a buried atmosphere, but are walking over hidden ponds and lakes and streams.

If you take a shallow basin and nearly fill it with sand, and then pour on to the sand about one third of the basinfull of water, the water will soon sink away, collecting for a certain depth at the bottom of the basin quite out of sight, but as really there, with its surface about as level as if there were no sand in the dish.   This represents the "ground water" of the soil.

Or, to put it in another way. Suppose you have a small lake in a hollow between the hills, fed by the rain-water which runs off from the adjoining slopes. If you fill this lake full of sand, so that the water is no longer visible, the lake is there all the same, but it has now become ground water instead of surface water, and is a type of the fixed subterranean sources of many of our water supplies. If the ground-water level lies just at the surface of the soil, remaining so for considerable periods, we have a swamp or bog.

For some distance above the level of the ground water the pores of the soil are more or less filled with water drawn up by capillary attraction. Most of the time in low or wooded regions, and after rains in dry, sandy countries, the pores all through the soil contain more or less moisture, which is carried out into the atmosphere with the tiny currents of ground air, spoken of above,—thus contributing by evaporation very largely at times to the aërial moisture which finally may gather in the clouds.

But we must look a little more closely at this ground water, which we should thoroughly understand, if we wish to study wells and springs intelligently by and by.

The soil layers over the earth's surface were largely deposited under the influence of water, which formed great seas and lakes, where now is land, and so the ruggedness of the solid rock surface is largely concealed. We can get little idea from the broad sweeps or gentle curves or swelling banks formed by the soil, of the hollows and jagged projections and uneven surfaces of the rock below.

Some idea of the ground water and its relations to various rock and soil layers may be obtained from a study of Fig. 1, which represents a section of the ground and underlying rock in a typical region. The water is indicated by the blue color.

Here is the primitive rock below, into which the water does not soak. This rock has been eroded or torn or worn away above, leaving rough sloping surfaces, in which are larger and smaller depressions. This whole region has been under water some time or other, for it is covered with rock detritus deposited in layers, gravel first, then sand. and over this the loam,

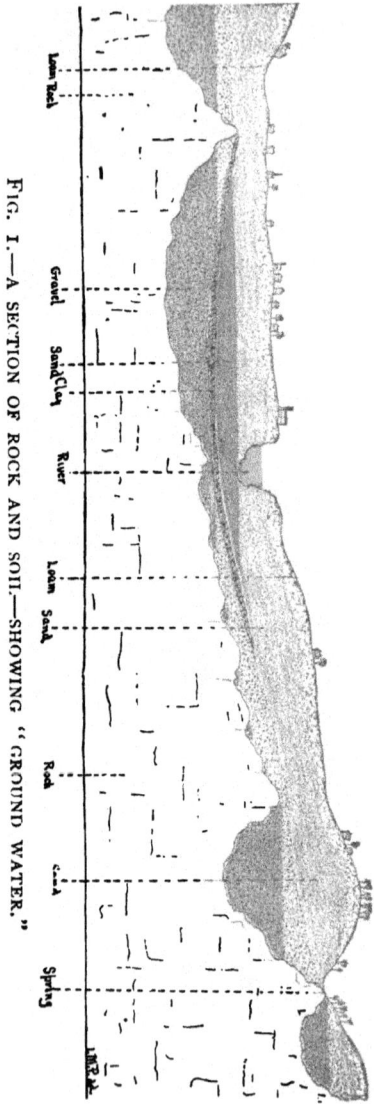

Fig. I.—A section of rock and soil—showing "ground water."

with its thin covering of vegetation. In the central portion of the region is a thin, impervious, somewhat basin-like clay bed, lying over the gravel. A river runs through the valley in a direction away from the observer. The smooth swelling contour of land gives no intimation of the roughness of the rock surfaces below.

It will be seen that the water which falls in rain on the hills at the right of the drawing will, when the hollows and subterranean lakes there are filled, run along down the sloping rock surface, entirely out of sight, as slowly flowing ground water, and finally collect in the valley, forming a deep subterranean reservoir in the gravel beds. It will further be observed that the rain which falls in the valley, in the region of the village, may be in part carried off by the river, in part soak into the sand layers and gather on the impervious clay bed, forming a reservoir of ground water above and entirely independent of the larger water mass below it. When the level of this clay-bed water is low, it may be reinforced from the river which flows just above it. When it is high, the water may run through the pores of the sand into the river and so be in part carried off.

It will be seen that the ground water comes to the surface at one point in the little valley on the high ground at the right, thus forming a spring, the overflow from which disappears directly in the sand and runs on to the lower level.

It is plain that the residents of the little village in the valley have four accessible sources of water supply for domestic use. The most obvious of these is the river. The next might be rain-water collected in cisterns. The next is from wells. Finally, if it were abundant enough there, the water might be brought in pipes from the spring on the hills some distance off to the right.

Now every resident in this village could get water by digging a well close to his house, except the one who unwittingly bought the land just over the mass of solid rock which rises above the ground water to the left of the middle of the picture. Some of these people would have to dig deeper wells than others, but all would sooner or later strike into the great subterranean reservoir largely fed from the adjacent hills.

The people who live over the clay bed could get water by digging comparatively shallow wells. But, as will be seen, the supply would not be large unless fed by the river, and, moreover, it would be water into which the drainage of the houses could readily pass. If they went a little deeper, however, piercing the clay bed, they would strike into the great supply.

This object-lesson will suffice to illustrate the more common subterranean sources of water supply. The wells and the springs, it will be seen, are after all supplied from the same sources, only in the one the water has to be dug for, while in the other, it comes spontaneously to the surface; or, as it would perhaps be more correct to say, the surface sinks to it.

In the so-called artesian wells from which the water gushes out, the ground water has found its way between two impervious strata and is kept here under pressure from the water crowding it from the sides, and so when a bore is made through the upper stratum, it comes gushing up. (See Fig. 2.) Sometimes these accumulations are very large, so that the water which is forced up may have found entrance between the impervious strata many miles away from the well. This is the case in the new artesian-well supply of the city of Memphis, Tenn. The water here enters the sand layers from forty to sixty miles away, and moves slowly along between impervious clay beds, filling, under pressure from the crowding water behind, the underground basin below the town.

The rate of flow of the ordinary ground water varies, of course, a good deal depending upon the porosity of the soil and the slope of the impervious surfaces, but in general it is very slow, averaging not much more, as a rule, than a foot an hour.

We are very apt to think that the volume of a river does not change much as it flows, except when visible tributary streams join it. But it very often happens that the slowly flowing ground water coming down unseen from the hills is pouring in its myriad tiny streams,

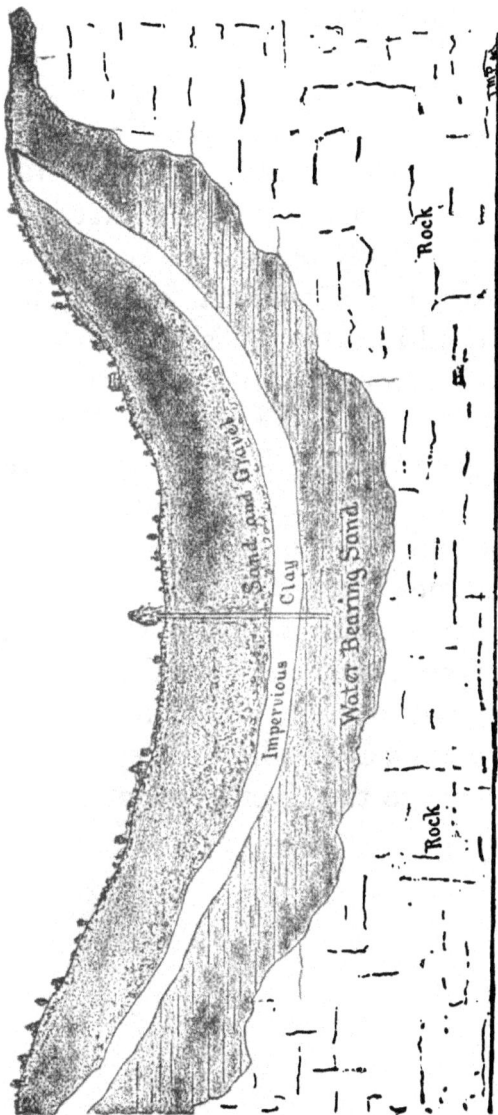

FIG. 2.—AN ARTESIAN WELL.

Sand and Gravel

Clay

Impervious

Water Bearing Sand

Rock

Rock

29

unseen because below the water level, in such aggregate amount as to greatly augment the river's volume from mile to mile. It not infrequently happens, however, that the banks and bed of a river become so tight and impervious, from the silt which little by little has been packed into the soil's pores, that it flows along as if in a trough through a veritable lake of ground water, and for long distances does not mingle with it. The ground water may, under these conditions, when the whole country slopes, be flowing on with its crawling current underneath the soil, side by side with the rushing river, with which it only mingles at last when both are merged into a larger stream. It even not infrequently happens that the ground water may in a limited region be flowing transversely to the river's flow at the surface.

CHAPTER V.

IF we could run a pipe far up into the air and draw our water from the clouds, we should be spared a world of trouble and annoyance. Up there is water distilled by the sun itself, and while it stays there it is just simple H_2O, pure enough to satisfy the atomic soul longings of the chemist himself.

But the moment it gets fairly condensed into available form and begins to fall through the air, especially in inhabited regions, it draws into solution more or less of the atmospheric gases, oxygen, nitrogen, and carbonic acid. It takes up, too, more complex chemical substances when they are present in the atmosphere, such as ammonia and various acids. As the rain-drops sweep through dusty air, they wash out of it and carry down with them the mul-

tifarious particles which compose the dust,
—bits of coal and soot, particles of iron and
stone and lime and various fabrics, tiny fragments of plants, and the numberless forms of
life, called germs, etc. All these foreign
things are gathered in when rain-water is collected in cisterns for household use.

When the water reaches the earth and
washes its more or less dirty surfaces and its
people, with their houses and streets and the
animals and plants, it takes up a good many
more impurities, notable among these being
the broken-down remnants of things once
alive, now called " organic matter." A portion
of this soiled water evaporates into the air,
leaving its dirt accumulations behind. A portion is taken up by plant rootlets, while the re-
mainder either clings in the pores of the soil,
or slowly sinks to deeper depths, until it
reaches the ground water.

Now, a very significant thing has been observed in regard to this water which sinks into
the soil charged with all kinds and all degrees
of foreign material, partly in solution, partly
in suspension. That is, that if the layers of
3

soil are thick enough and of the right kinds, and if the water passes slowly enough through it, by the time it reaches the ground-water reservoir, it may have largely freed itself of its foreign burdens, and joins its kin below in pure and wholesome form. The water while on the earth's surface may be of a very disagreeable color and odor ; it may contain many chemical substances of most undesirable nature, and whole hordes of minute living things. But by the time it reaches the ground water, it may have lost nearly all of the foreign chemical substances and all of its suspended matters, so efficient are the complex physical and chemical processes which in the earth's great underground laboratory are ceaselessly going on.

This is called natural filtration, and is one of those great processes by which in far-reaching cycles Mother Earth renovates her limited stock of life-stuff, and so keeps her children supplied always with the best. When, however, her pet nursling, man, puts his careless or ignorant or meddling finger into the machinery and disturbs the regular course of things by crowding too much filthy material into one place, or by drawing too heavily upon the supplies which should slowly accumulate, or by cutting off the forests which shelter large regions from too rapid water losses, he is very apt to find that he has upset the balance of things and usually suffers for it, sooner or later, by those personal punishments for ignorance or folly, which we call disease.

A great deal of thought and research have been expended in trying to make out the nature and details of this marvellous cleansing power of the soil. Aside from the more obvious alterations in the chemical constitution of the foreign ingredients of the water, the chemists used to be disposed to sum up the nature of the process by saying,—oxidation. This was very well for its time, but we shall presently see that a very subtle and very curious agency is at work here, which until recently has been nearly wholly ignored.

It happens in many regions that the water, as it soaks into the earth or runs over the rocks, not only gives up some of its foreign ingredients, but actually takes up others. In this way, water may take up mineral substances which make it what we call "hard," in distinction from rain-water and most surface waters, which are "soft."

Let us now run hastily over the different sources of water supply, and note in a general way their qualities under the usual conditions.

Rain-water in the open country may be very pure and good. But in towns or in the vicinity of certain manufactories, rain-water collected in cisterns is usually not very good for drinking and cooking purposes, unless it be in some way artificially purified.

The ground water in most regions, particularly if it is situated at some distance beneath the surface, so that it has been purified by ground filtration, is naturally and usually good. The deeper water, such as is stored in the great underground reservoirs and comes up in artesian wells and in the varied mineral and other deep springs, is reckoned as one of the purest sources of supply.

The purity of surface waters, such as those of lakes and pools and streams, depends very much upon the region from which they are fed, and especially upon the behavior and intelligence of the people who live near their borders. They may be said to naturally furnish good water, although in the case of rivers, foreign material, such as clay and other fine particles, may at all times, or at certain periods of the year, be washed in in such quantities as to make the water turbid, and so greatly interfere with its attractiveness, if they do not make it actually unwholesome.

The great trouble with rivers, and more or less with lakes, is, that in their vicinity people are very apt to settle and build cities and towns and dwellings, and the sewage and other waste of these residences are apt very naturally but very wickedly, to be allowed to run directly into the waters, thus polluting them, if not for the sinners themselves, in rivers at least, for their neighbors down the stream.

We shall be obliged, disagreeable as the subject is, to look a little more closely by and by into the various ways in which man becomes his own worst enemy by rendering fairly unfit for use those sources of water supply which Nature has so bountifully and so perfectly adapted to the uses of the clean but not the dirty dwellers in her domain. But before we do this, we must try to gain a little clearer insight into the way in which by natural filtration the great underground sources are kept clean and pure.

CHAPTER VI.

A STUDY OF THE LIVING EARTH.

WHEN we have learned what we can of the nature and extent and movements of the buried atmosphere, and of the hidden lakes and ponds and streams, and of their multitudinous feeders trickling through the soil, we might seem to have exhausted the story of this subterranean activity, changing with the winds and rains and dew-falls and with the alternations of the seasons and the days and nights. But the most curious and complex phases of the story are yet to come.

We cannot consider here the vast and ceaseless changes which are going on in the soil under the influence of plant roots and of various underground animals, especially of worms, though these might well form a chapter in the story of the living earth. We will also tarry here only to allude to the varied chemical combinations and decompositions which go on in the soil between the foreign substances in the water and the soil ingredients as the water trickles among them.

It is estimated that in a cubical mass of fine sand about three feet on a side, the aggregate free surfaces of all the sand particles may amount to many thousand square feet. But it would take us into too intricate a subject were we to dwell upon the curious and powerful physical effects, upon the water and its ingredients, of these enormous aggregate surfaces of the soil particles. By means of these large surfaces they are able to attract to themselves thin sheets of the water, and thus expose it to the action of the oxygen of the ground air, or in other ways to separate and retain or destroy foreign substances, even those in solution, such as coloring materials and various poisons, and many kinds of organic matter.

By organic substances we mean materials which have once formed a part of some living thing, animal or plant, but are now dead and ready in Nature's cycle to be resolved into sim-

pler combinations fit to be used again. These
organic materials which the soil filtration re-
moves from the water, contain, as a rule, a
good deal of carbon and nitrogen and hydrogen in varied combinations. These are apt to
be torn asunder and separated from their
other constituents and recombined in the form
of new-formed water, carbonic acid, and nitric
or some closely allied acids, which again may
enter into new liaisons without delay. This
disposal of the nitrogen of the old dead organic matter, by its conversion into new oxy-
genated compounds, is called "nitrification,"
and is one of the most important cleansing
processes which goes on in nature.

We can readily enough understand how, by
straining dirty water through the soil, most of
the substances held in suspension might be
removed. We can readily assent, as a temporary hypothesis, to the conjecture that the
more complex changes to which we have al-
luded, such as the chemical decomposition and
recombinations of the elements of organic
matter might in some way be explained by
their oxidation when exposed over the enor-

mous aggregate surface of the soil particles. In fact, this general view was held to be measurably satisfactory for a long time.

But after a while the restless souls of the chemists and biologists became dissatisfied with such a general explanation of so important a process. They, moreover, fell upon some observations which seemed to indicate that there might be something more in the matter.

It occurred to somebody once to test the water-cleansing capacity of a selected volume of soil in the laboratory. When this had been done, the same soil was heated up very hot, so that if there were any living things in it they would, said the experimenter, certainly have been killed. When the soil had cooled, he tested its cleansing powers for dirty water again, and found that they had been largely annihilated. The sand and gravel acted as a strainer still, and separated the coarser impurities from the water, but these more complex and, on the whole, much more important changes in organic matter did not occur.

Now, why was this? Here in the soil were the same solid particles unchanged, the same enormous surfaces, the same sort of air-filled pores, but the water was not purified as it was before the heating of the soil. This matter is worth looking into, because it involves some facts which we must very thoroughly understand if we are going to become intelligent judges of the water supplies of our households.

A good while before these observations had been made on the effects of heating the soil, scientific men had been exploring a new world of life among organisms, which are so minute that they lie far beyond the range of the unaided vision,—I mean the bacteria. These and their modes of study have already been described in sufficient detail for our purposes in two other books of this little series,[1] to which I must refer.

It will be sufficient to say here that these tiny organisms can be readily cultivated artificially in the laboratory. If one takes any of the substances which contain them, or to which they cling, as earth, air, water, and nearly every other solid thing in inhabited regions, as

[1] " The Story of the Bacteria," " Dust and Its Dangers."

well as the bodies of men and animals, and mixes portions of them with a little specially prepared bacterial food, these organisms will grow, and can be separated into species in tubes each by itself, and the life history of each form followed out in detail.

The more common and useful of the methods employed in studying the bacteria now are those devised and formulated more than a decade ago by Dr. Robert Koch, of Berlin, whose great achievements in this and allied fields are to-day so widely known and valued.

Soon after the introduction of these methods of studying the minute forms of vegetable life, students in this new field went scurrying hither and yon with their prying tests, and when it occurred to some of them to see what a little common field earth had to show, and they planted a few tiny fragments of this earth-wreckage by scattering its particles through a little of the prepared bacterial or germ food, they found, after a couple of days, that wherever a tiny particle of the soil had lain there had grown a perfectly colossal number of little plant masses, each from a single germ. When these early observers had recovered from their surprise at finding that the soil was fairly swarming with these invisible living germs, they took measured amounts of the earth, and found that not infrequently in a mass of earth no bigger than a pea there might be many millions of living germs. Some are moulds, some yeasts, but they are mostly bacteria of many kinds.

It was also learned that while these minute invisible germs were everywhere very abundant in the soil, the number varied a good deal in different places. It was further found, and this is a very significant thing, that in general the number of living germs diminishes as we go downward in the soil, until finally we find in most regions that at a depth which varies from three to five feet they cease to be present in any considerable number, or are absent altogether. Of course if the soil has been recently disturbed to a considerable depth, or if it be frequently flooded with dirty water or sewage, or other organic refuse, the depths at which these germs are found may be much greater than those mentioned as usual.

But what has all this to do, you say, with the purification of water by the soil. Bacteria and other germs are among the forms of dirt in the water which are to be removed by soil filtration. What can they have to do with the purification process ? Is it possible that they will kill one another in the soil, and feed upon and thus destroy in its harmful shape the dead and poisonous organic matter of the water? Yes, these are just some of the performances which these invisible friends of man have been trained into through the long cycles which ushered in his geologic age.

In feeding and growing, the bacteria tear apart organic matter of various kinds. A part of the material thus released from its former combinations is assimilated by the bacteria themselves ; a part is set free to share in any new chemical adventure which the vicissitudes of time and place and season may sanction.

In their life processes, the bacteria may set free materials which are different for each species, and which are varied in their effects upon other living things. Some of these freed materials do no harm, either to the germs which elaborate them or to any other living things. Some of them, on the other hand, may when they are present, even in very minute amounts, poison and kill either the germs which formed them or other species.

Now recent experiments have shown that there may be an enormous destruction of germs of one kind or another in the soil, under certain conditions ; so that even sewage-water, containing millions of living germs to every pint, if poured on a limited portion of soil *under proper conditions*, year in, year out, may come out below clear and practically free from germs ; while, as examinations show, the number of living germs in the soil used as a filter does not increase beyond a certain point.

In the hodgepodge of new chemical materials, which are produced in fluids which contain many species of bacteria growing together, it is difficult to say very much about the exact nature of these different new and sometimes poisonous substances, but that they act to continually destroy some of the germs is pretty well ascertained.

CHAPTER VII.

THE LIVING EARTH.—(*Concluded.*)

LET us now see if we can bring a little order out of this apparently chaotic condition of affairs in the purification of water as it trickles through the soil. The facts are that we may start with water soaking into the surface, which contains not only large numbers of exceedingly minute bacteria and other germs, and various organic and inorganic suspended particles, but holds in actual solution organic and other foreign materials. At the end of the soil filtration, the water, as it reaches its resting-place in the ground-water reservoirs, may contain no bacteria, no suspended particles of any kind, and no organic matter in solution. Its only foreign ingredients may be small amounts of inorganic compounds, of no special practical importance.

Great light has been thrown on this problem by carefully conducted experiments on limited quantities of soil or sand, subjected to conditions as nearly akin as might be to those of natural filtration.

In the first place, it has been found that if one starts with an artificial filter-bed of perfectly clean sand, containing no bacteria, and floods it with dirty water, the water which comes through for the first few days and for a much longer time, if the weather be cold, will be but little if at all purified. Its coarser suspended particles may have been caught in the sand pores, and so it may be clearer, but its dissolved organic matter and its bacteria may not be at all diminished. Indeed for some time, strange as it may appear, the numbers of the bacteria may have largely increased. In fact, it appears that the pores of such a fresh sand-filter with the organic matter suspended in the water form a most excellent breeding-place for bacteria.

This seems discouraging. But let the experiment go on, and after a while if the dirty water has not been forced through the sand too fast, it will be found that the number of living germs which come out in the water at the bottom is growing steadily smaller, and finally the water may be nearly or quite germ-free. Now if the chemist exposes some of the filtered water to his delicate tests, he may find that the organic matter which was in solution in the water at the top has already diminished or entirely disappeared, being represented perhaps by nitrogen, which has formed harmless combinations with oxygen.

It really seems as if the more living, growing bacteria you had in the upper layers of your filter-bed, the freer became the water below, both of bacteria and organic matter. This is, in fact, the case. We do in this experiment what nature does on the large scale,—make the bacteria fight the organic matter and themselves.

But how is this effect produced? The bacteria are so small that hundreds of them could easily pass abreast through the smallest spaces between the sand particles. What holds them back?

When the sand particles at the upper portion of these filter-beds have been carefully examined, it has been found that they are, after a few days, completely encased in a slimy gelatin-like envelope, formed of a material which many bacteria secrete around themselves as they grow. This bacteria-formed slime more or less fills the pores of the filter-bed enclosing the bacteria themselves and the sand particles, and catches and holds fast on its sticky surfaces, not only suspended matter of various kinds, but the new bacteria which come on to the filter and start to work their way down through its pores. Here many of them, like good prisoners, set to work to make the best of the situation, and if their nature permits, turn to and help to make more of this trap-slime to capture the next comers.

Many of the entangled germs, however, do not form this material, and these may die in large numbers where they lie. On the other hand, this enforced detention is simply paradise for many of the germs. Here they are, resting at ease in a slimy confinement, with boundless supplies of just the food they want slowly trickling by them. This food is dead organic matter, which the average bacterium simply dotes on and recks little whether it be in solid form or in solution, so there be enough of it. At it he goes then, and by some wholly inscrutable phase of the life power in his tiny body, asunder fall the atoms which have once been parts of animal or plant. That part which the tiny life spark needs to keep its glow a-going is appropriated. The rest it leaves, its atomic cravings unsatisfied, and only too ready to succumb to the wiles of the ever-amorous oxygen, which must always be present in a perfectly acting filter-bed.

The slowness and the intermittent character of natural soil filtration is a very important matter in the accomplishment of perfect results, because in the times between the rains, the soil pores have a chance to become filled with stores of oxygen, in the form of ground air.

Behold now the secret of this marvellous alembic into which may go things most foul and harmful, but out of which comes the very type of purity and cleanliness—clear spring water. It is largely the bacteria, living, growing, multiplying, following their life impulses silently and unseen, each after its kind, which, supported by the active agency of oxygen, bring about this beneficent result. And this goes on, not alone at the behest of the experimenter, but over the whole wide domain of nature, where water more or less impure falls upon the rock-ruins of the earth crust and slowly makes its way to the capacious bosom of the earth through the bacteria-laden upper-soil layers.

Now it may be that this sounds very fantastical, not to say nonsensical, but it is an accurate description, only in simple language, of some of those things which we already know about the purifying agencies of the soil. These little workmen, the bacteria, are, in this domain at least, our benefactors, and we should do them the justice to acknowledge it. There are black sheep among them, but these fellows delving for us in the soil are assuredly the whitest of the white.

We are slowly making headway in the knowledge of the individual species of bacteria which carry on this work for us, and already expert and sagacious workers, both in this country and abroad, are describing and studying the life history and naming some of those particular species which are active in disposing of the organic nitrogen in impure water and the soil. There is already a well-known class of " nitrifying bacteria."

We shall recur briefly to this subject when we come to consider the methods for artificial purification of water for domestic use. But now, even, it would seem, when we glance back at these curious and in the aggregate colossal doings of the myriad of tiny plants in the soil, that we were not too fanciful in entitling this long chapter " A Study of the Living Earth."

CHAPTER VIII.

SOME WATER IMPURITIES.

IT is not necessary that water should be chemically pure in order to be good for the more important domestic uses, such as cooking and drinking. In fact, no natural water is wholly free from some foreign ingredients. We say, in general, that a good water should be transparent, colorless, odorless, and tasteless, and should, on standing, deposit no sediment. But water may fulfil all these conditions and still not be fit for domestic use, because some of the most objectionable things which water may contain are wholly imperceptible to the unaided senses. I do not purpose to speak here in detail of the mineral substances which water may contain, dissolved out of rocks, and which may make it what is called " hard," or be present in such form and quantity as to constitute a so-called mineral water, but only of those materials which may fairly be called impurities, and thus may have a bearing upon the salubrity of the water.

We may conveniently divide the important impurities of water into two groups : first, those which are not living ; and second, those which are alive.

1. If we look first at those impurities which are not alive, we find that these may be either mineral substances in the form of particles or in solution, or they may be organic substances, also in the form of particles or in solution.

Mineral substances in the form of particles in water, if in considerable quantities, as in the water of rivers running through a clay country, make the water so uninviting in appearance that people are very apt to get rid of them by some method of straining the water, and so we need say no more about them. Mineral substances in solution in water may, as in the true mineral waters, be of certain medicinal uses, and do not constitute, as we have said, real impurities.

But there are inorganic compounds which

the chemist finds in water, which, although not in themselves at all harmful to the consumer, indicate that there have been in the water a class of substances which are of serious import. For example, except in certain regions, common salt in considerable amount does not belong in good water, nor does nitric acid and the nitrates and nitrites, which are formed from the oxidation of organic matter, nor do salts of ammonia. Some of these things are found naturally in certain regions, and then their presence is not of importance. They are in themselves, furthermore, not harmful to the consumer. Their significance, under ordinary circumstances, is this : they usually indicate that the water has been polluted with sewage or with some form of dead organic matter ; that such pollution is possible, and hence, although at the moment of analysis dangerous sewage or dangerous organic matter may not be present, it may presumably at any time get into the water source again. These substances are, as we say, symptomatic of more or less dangerous pollution.

Dead organic matter, although not always harmful in small quantities, is matter which may be undergoing putrefaction, and hence is always regarded, when present in water in considerable amounts, as an objectionable ingredient.

We cannot enter here into the details of analysis and conclusion upon which the chemist bases his judgment of the character of a given specimen of drinking-water, because this is not the special line of study which we are following in this book. But we may say in brief that when the chemist finds in the water dead organic matter, either in the form of particles, or in solution in considerable quantities, or when he finds such chemical compounds as indicate that such organic matter has been there when it ought not to be, his suspicion is aroused as to the salubrity of the water, and he must investigate its source. If he finds that it comes from such sources as indicate a pollution with human or animal waste, the water must be condemned, because the door is probably, if not certainly, open through which disease-producing agencies may enter.

It will be seen that the chemist in his examinations of water does not, for the most part, get his finger upon the actual causes of disease in dangerous water, but finds only those telltale traces of materials which often accompany disease-producing stuff.   It should not be inferred from this that the examinations of the chemist are unimportant, because it not infrequently happens that in no other way than by his analysis can we get an indication of dangerous agents in water.

2. We come now to the living impurities in water.   These again we find to be of two classes : first, animals ; and second, plants. We speak here, of course, only of the minute forms of life in water.   The tiny animals which may be present in ordinary drinking-water in comparatively small numbers belong largely among the so-called protozoa, or simple forms of animal life, and are, so far as we know, of no importance whatsoever in their relationship to health, and we need therefore give no further thought to them.   Very impure water may, however, contain the eggs of certain animal parasites, which we cannot now consider.

With the minute plants, however, which water may contain, the case is different, for in this group of living things are certain forms occasionally finding their way into drinking-water which are capable of inducing serious and even fatal disease.

There are certain moss-like growths, called algæ, which occasionally get into reservoirs of water and grow very rapidly, and so do harm either by blocking up the pipes or filling the reservoirs, or by a rapid decomposition, which gives the water a very bad taste or smell and so makes it unfit for use. These forms we will not further consider.

We come at last to the great group of minute plants called *bacteria*, towards which our rapid survey of this field has been leading us. But here let us stop a moment to correct a false impression which the name *bacteria* nearly always makes when spoken in connection with things which we use as food.

It is very unfortunate that the earliest notions which people nowadays get of these minute living things should usually be associated with their relationship to disease. So

that in the minds of most people who have
been hearing about bacteria, now and then,
and especially often quite recently, the name
bacteria is associated with some horrid conception of a deadly being, like a bug or worm,
which burrows or gnaws its way into the body
and works havoc there. Now the sooner anybody who is in this condition gets out of it, the
better will it be for his peace of mind. For
the knowledge of these unseen fellow-dwellers
with us on the earth has come to stay, and a
large part of the mental inquietude which
people have about them is due to mistaken
notions as to their nature and importance.

Because one knows that tigers are ferocious,
he does n't shudder whenever any member of
the feline tribe is mentioned. Because some
plants are poisonous, we don't think that we
must have recourse to an exclusive meat diet ;
nor need we when bacteria are named forthwith imagine that a medical theme is on the
carpet. Of the thousands of bacteria which
are teeming everywhere about us, even in
the cleanest of inhabited places, it is but an
insignificant number whose relationships to

man are any thing but beneficent or indifferent.

The species which do harm are, so far as we know, very few, and so associated with the persons or animals who are suffering from the diseases which they induce that if only a reasonable degree of intelligent cleanliness be exercised our risks of coming in contact with them are very slight indeed. The fact is then that the sooner we get a fair amount of knowledge about these tiny organisms, so that we can incorporate a reasonable cleanliness into our routine, the sooner can we go singing on our way with that freedom from apprehension which belonged to the pre-bacterial epoch ; a freedom, too, enhanced by the consciousness that intelligently clean rooms and houses, cities and food, mean a larger degree of immunity from many forms of serious disease.

It follows from this rather long and rambling plea for justice to the mild-mannered members of the ubiquitous germ fraternity, that we need not be disturbed in the least when we see in some book or journal that Prof. A. has found 800 germs in a thimbleful of city drinking-water, or that Dr. B. estimates that there are at least a million in a schooner of beer. All this is of no personal significance whatsoever to us, except as a more or less interesting fact in nature, *unless*—please note this well—unless the aforesaid gentlemen show in their case reason to believe that these same multitudinous waifs belong among the harmful members of the germ fraternity, or in some way foreshadow the actual or possible presence of these.

There are indeed, as I have intimated, some very stern realities associated with a few species of bacteria. But they need not overshadow existence, even in crowded towns, if we but live up to the light which science is throwing wide abroad in this domain, and do not permit the sanitary affairs of our municipalities to fall into the clutches of mercenary political tricksters. If we do this we deserve such mental inquietude as will the sooner incite us to compel reform.

CHAPTER IX.

THE UNSEEN WATER FLORA.

WE return now to the bacteria which are present in varying numbers in nearly all surface water and in much of the ground water which does not lie buried at considerable depths.

More than a hundred different species of bacteria found in water have been described. Many of these have been named and their individual life histories studied out. It is a very curious and motley group, these unseen water-dwellers, when we get them growing in the laboratory so that we can see them.

A good many of them are mobile and under the microscope may be seen darting about wildly and apparently aimlessly. Many of them form brilliant colors when under artificial cultivation. Some are phosphorescent. Many of the water bacteria are lovers of oxygen, and thus around air bubbles there is often a great gathering of the clans.   Others seem to have as persistent, not to say malignant, a hatred of oxygen as has the average theatre proprietor, and thrive best, as he often seems to do, far from this popular gas.

Many species dread the light, and sulk or pine and die in the sun's rays.   Almost all forms take kindly to mild temperatures, however, and if they find a good warm nook not too sunny, with plenty of old plant ruins in it, they must be as happy as bacteria can be, in a world so largely given over to their betters.

The bacteria are rarely uniformly distributed through a mass of water, the centre of population constantly changing.   In lakes and ponds there are more, as a rule, near the shores than in the central deeper parts, very likely because near the shores there is more food and usually a more congenial temperature. The currents in rivers, however, largely overweigh the individual preferences of the germs as to their locations.   They are, as a rule, considerably more abundant in most waters in summer time than in winter.

Very few of them when present in the moderate numbers which are found in clean natural waters produce ill effects when taken into the body in drinking-water. They are of no more significance as articles of consumption, because they are alive, than are the tiny living cells which make up in myriads all of the fresh vegetable foods which we consume. So there is no intrinsic reason whatsoever why one should be more sensitive about the few thousands of living bacterial cells which he may take into his system in a glass of water, than he is about the thousands of living cells which he consumes when he eats an apple or a plate of salad.

There are certain species of bacteria which seem especially to belong in water, for we find them in natural water from the most widely separated parts of the earth. Many forms grow readily, and multiply with incredible rapidity in the purest of water, producing in a short time such enormous numbers that it is difficult to see where they get material enough

5

to feed upon. Such forms are called *par excellence* "water bacteria." It appears that many forms are cannibals, consuming the bodies of their defunct brethren.

One very naturally questions how it is that bacteria get into so many natural waters, since the cloud water does not contain them, and the deep, well filtered ground water is largely free.

Moderate numbers of germs are, as we have seen, caught from the floating dust in the rain-drops as they fall, and these in regions where there is not good ground filtration may stay there until the water is collected in streams and lakes. Then the soil, whose superficial layers are, as we have seen, usually swarming with them, is washed off more or less from the shores into streams and lakes by rains, and large numbers are often set free by erosion of the banks. The soil is thus, on the one hand, the great purifier of water from its bacterial ingredients by filtration ; and, on the other, is one of the great suppliers of them from the banks of still or running reservoirs.

In settled regions human habitations and certain industries form one of the greatest and

most significant sources of the bacterial impurities of water, since, as we have already
seen, sewage and other bacteria-laden waste is
very apt to be run off into the great natural
sources of water supply. We see at once that
human and animal waste, especially the former,
furnishes the most significant source of bacterial water pollution, because in this we are
most apt to have the species of bacteria which
have caused disease, and may again, if they
but gain access to the bodies of the water
consumers.

When men first began to study the bacteria
systematically by the new technique, everybody thought, just as most people do still, that
as serious disease could be caused by bacteria,
the presence of germs of all kinds in water,
even in moderate numbers, might be of sanitary importance. But since we have learned
to discriminate between harmful and harmless
species, and since we have learned that a certain number fairly belong in water, our views
as to their significance have materially changed.
We no longer ask whether there are any bacteria in a given specimen of drinking-water, but

whether there are so many and of such forms as to justify the suspicion that there has been a pollution of the water from a source which could furnish the dangerous kinds.

It is, however, probable that exceedingly large numbers of the ordinarily harmless species may in especially sensitive persons, such as young children, give rise to important disorders of the digestive system. But of this we know too little yet to speak very definitely.

CHAPTER X.

A WATER CENSUS.

I T will thus be evident that it is of a good deal of importance to find out by a bacterial analysis of the greatest variety of natural waters, from the most varied regions, what, on the whole, is to be considered as a fair number of these germs which water may contain and still be regarded as salubrious. In other words, it is desirable to establish what may be called the *bacterial norm* of good drinking-water.

Now this might be thought a very simple matter, requiring only a diligent examination of water from all possible sources. And such at first it was deemed to be. But very soon after scientific men got to work in this field, difficulties began to crop out which made the problem seem a more and more complex one.

It was found that many deep springs and wells and many mountain streams and some lakes were practically germ-free.   On the other hand, it was shown that not infrequently springs and wells and streams whose water, by experience and from inspection, appeared of the best quality, might contain a good many living germs.   The influence of stagnation and temperature and exposure to air and light, and many other factors, must, it would seem, be taken into the account.

A series of examinations of the water in Paris by Miquel gave the following interesting results.   The rain-water in a park just outside of the city contained, on the average, 4 living bacteria to a cubic centimetre (that is, to about one third of a teaspoonful).   The rain-water in the city contained 17.   The water of the Seine, just above Paris, contained 300 bacteria, while within the city, after receiving the contents of the sewers, there were 200,000, to one cubic centimetre.   The river water, which had been used in the floating laundries, which form such familiar features along the banks of the Seine, in Paris, was found to contain

26,000,000 living germs to one cubic centimetre.

The river Spree, which runs through the
city of Berlin, was found on one occasion to
contain above the city 82,000 germs, while
below it showed 10,180,000, to one cubic centimetre. These figures show what the bacterial contents of greatly polluted rivers may
be.

On the other hand, the river Rhone, at the
point from which the Geneva water supply is
taken, has been found to contain only from
24 to 75 bacteria to one cubic centimetre.

The Hudson River water above Albany was
found to contain on two occasions a little over
2,000 bacteria to one cubic centimetre.

The Potomac River water at Washington
has been found by Smith to contain, at various seasons of the year, all the way from 75
to 3,774 bacteria to a cubic centimetre.

Unpolluted streams and lakes contain, as a
rule, very much smaller numbers of germs
than those which have been mentioned.

The writer has made a series of several
hundreds of bacterial analyses of the unfil-

tered Croton water, as delivered through the
pipes in the city of New York, at all months
in the year except June, July, and August,
extending from 1886 to 1890. The highest
numbers of bacteria are almost invariably
found after rains or the melting of the snow
in the spring, and more recently, after the
commencement of the use of, or after changes
in, the new aqueduct. The largest number
ever found was 1,950 to one cubic centimetre;
the lowest, 20. Counting up the results of all
the analyses of the Croton made during this
period, the average number, up to December,
1890, is 319.

The number of bacteria in the ordinary well
waters varies a great deal, both with and without evidences of gross pollution. In some
regions there are always more than in others.
The freedom of well waters from bacteria depends primarily upon the efficiency of the
natural filtration and the resulting purity of
the ground water. But if the water is stag-
nant, so that the bacteria which naturally live
in water can increase in number, and very little is drawn out ; if contaminations are allowed

to enter from the sides or top of the well, the number of germs will, as would be expected, be usually large.

The effect of drawing out large volumes of water from a well and allowing it to refill from the ground supply is often very remarkable in reducing for a time the number of the bacteria. This is because the incoming water is filtered ground water. But if an examination of the water which enters the well immediately after the old bacteria-laden supply has been drawn shows large numbers of germs, the inference is justified that the ground water is impure.

Many thousands of analyses of all sorts of water have been made, and, on the whole, we feel that we can say that good, unpolluted natural waters may contain, on the average, all the way from none to five hundred bacteria to one cubic centimetre. If there are more than this, it becomes desirable to look into the sources of the water and see if we can account for the excess by any unobjectionable natural conditions. If we can, a few hundreds, more or less, does not seem to be of serious import.

But, on the other hand, if the study of the water sources to which our analyses have directed us show us a possibility of explaining the excess by a direct or indirect pollution with sewage or other human or animal waste, then the water must be condemned, for at such pollution the line must be drawn at all hazards, if we would avoid the possibility or probability of incurring bacterial disease. Nay, more than this. Though at the moment of examination the water be as free from germs as cloud vapor itself, if it is found to be polluted by sewage or other human or animal waste, it should be condemned out of hand. That way danger lies.

The opinion which the bacteriologist forms of water after its analysis depends, however, not alone on the number of living germs which it contains, but also on the variety of species which are present. This is important, because it often happens that the simple multiplication in water of the harmless " water bacteria " may give rise to large numbers of one or two harmless species. But in sewer water and in human and animal waste there are usually many different species, so that a water which contains many forms of bacteria may be more indicative of serious pollution than one which contains more germs of one or few kinds.

But, it may be asked, does not water purify itself after a while in large lakes or in running streams, so that though at some points considerable pollution takes place, at others in the same source it may be free from danger? There is no doubt that there is such a thing as natural or spontaneous purification of sewage-polluted water, apart from filtration in the soil or aërial evaporation. But we should be very guarded in our confidence in the extent to which this occurs, at least until we know more definitely about it.

A good deal of the current belief as to the so-called spontaneous purification of water rests upon the facts which were gathered from chemical examinations before we knew of the significance, or even the existence, of bacteria in water, and before we knew of the relationship between certain bacteria and disease. The chemists found, indeed, that in water which contained large amounts of objectionable organic matter from sewage poured into a running stream, this might practically disappear after exposure to the air and other influences. But even their most delicate analyses are too crude to take cognizance of the bacteria, which, after all, are of the greatest practical significance. The bacteria are living things, and it is n't always necessary to have a fixed amount, or number, of them to produce disease, when other conditions are favorable, as it is with poisons which are not self-propagating.

Dilution of sewage, of course, diminishes, in direct proportion to its amount, the chances of the consumer of the water getting any of the dangerous germs. But that leaves an unpleasant possibility of evil, and does not remove the essential filthiness of the condition.

In fact, it may be said in general that the number of bacteria in sewage-polluted streams does diminish in one way or another, which we have not the space to go into here, as the water flows farther and farther from the polluting source. But, on the whole, considering the possible danger and the absolute filthiness of drinking even diluted sewage, the only rational course, as it seems to the writer, is either to prevent the entrance of sewage into sources of water-supply, by stringent legal enactments, or, if this cannot be wholly done, to adopt for such waters some artificial methods of purification on the large scale. Of these we shall speak presently.

CHAPTER XI.

SOME WAYS OF GETTING WATER.

THE ways in which water is stored and distributed on a large scale for use in towns, we shall not dwell upon here, because this book is designed rather for the individual householder than for those intrusted with the interests of many people. We will, in fact, consider only the means by which people gain access to the ground-water supplies, because this, after all, is the greatest and most widespread source.

First, a glance at springs. There is a general impression, most fondly cherished, that wherever water runs out of the earth on to the surface it is pure and wholesome. This is in many cases true, in many cases wholly false. We have seen that spring water is in general just the same thing as ground water, only it makes its appearance at the surface in natural springs, without being dug for. Spring water then is exposed to the same contaminating and the same purifying agencies as other ground water. We do not now speak of mineral and hot springs, which may have origin very deep in the earth, and draw their supplies from far-distant and complex sources.

We must remember that there is no especial mystery about the water which we dig for in the earth or which gushes up spontaneously in the ordinary springs. It may come to us, indeed, clear, sparkling, cool, out of the dark recesses of the earth, as if new-created for our use, but it is mostly the same old water which shared in the rainbow's arches, pattered on the leaves, or swept the surface of the ground in torrents—yesterday, last week, last month, last year. In the great alembic it has been purified and perhaps, indeed, partly re-created out of elemental combinations, torn apart in the recesses of the soil.

In uninhabited regions, in the forests, wherever excessive contaminations of the soil with human or animal or manufacturing waste do not occur, we may fairly assume that the ground water from springs is wholesome and one of the best forms in which we can get it. But the moment we introduce human habitations, with their multitudinous forms of waste, with their soiled cleansing-water with their animal attachés, all pouring filth into the soil in limited areas, it frequently happens that the balance is destroyed and the ground water becomes contaminated, not only with organic matter of unwholesome character, but may become bacteria-laden as well.

When such not only unpurified but actually contaminated ground water gushes out in the form of a spring, it is often used by otherwise very sensible people, although it may not look very good and may taste very bad, just because it is spring water; and spring water, as they have been taught, must be good water. Now when any such condition as this is suspected, it is n't always necessary to run to the chemist or to the bacteriologist to have an analysis made. A careful inspection of the surroundings of the spring; an attentive study of the probable source of the water which comes to

the light here ; an heroic effort to get out of
the thrall of the word spring, and a moderate
use of common-sense will, in nine cases out of
ten, do more to set the spring's owner or user
right as to its merits or demerits, than would
the analyses of the whole Faculty.

One great difficulty with springs in inhabited
regions is that they are not properly protected
from surface contaminations.

Let us now turn to those means by which
the concealed ground water is brought to light
in what are called wells. The typical old-
fashioned well almost everybody is familiar
with, especially in the older parts of this
country. A deep hole is dug in the ground,
in what seems to the local expert a promising
region, or, as is most often the case, at as short
a distance as practicable from the house and
barn and other necessary outhouses. When
water is struck—that is, when the diggers
have got down to the ground water, the sides
of the hole are stoned or bricked up, a plat-
form is laid, and a curb with some sort of
hoisting apparatus is placed around the opening.

More recently it is often found better to

6

drive an iron tube, a few inches in diameter, down through the soil layers until the ground water is reached. The tube has a solid point to pierce the soil as it goes down, and at its lower end is a series of small openings through which the ground water can enter the tube. The water is drawn out of the tube by a pump. These are called driven wells. See Fig. 3.

When a large amount of water is to be drawn from the ground-water supply, a series of large perforated pipes are often laid down in the soil below the level of the ground water. These all communicate with a great central tube or chamber, from which the water is pumped as it flows in from the numerous feeders radiating off in all directions.

All of these forms of wells are, as will be seen, simply means of draining the ground water into open spaces in the soil from which it may be readily raised. All properly constructed wells are so situated that the soil forms a great natural filter about them, and upon the maintenance of this soil-filter in perfect working order depends the purity of the water obtained.

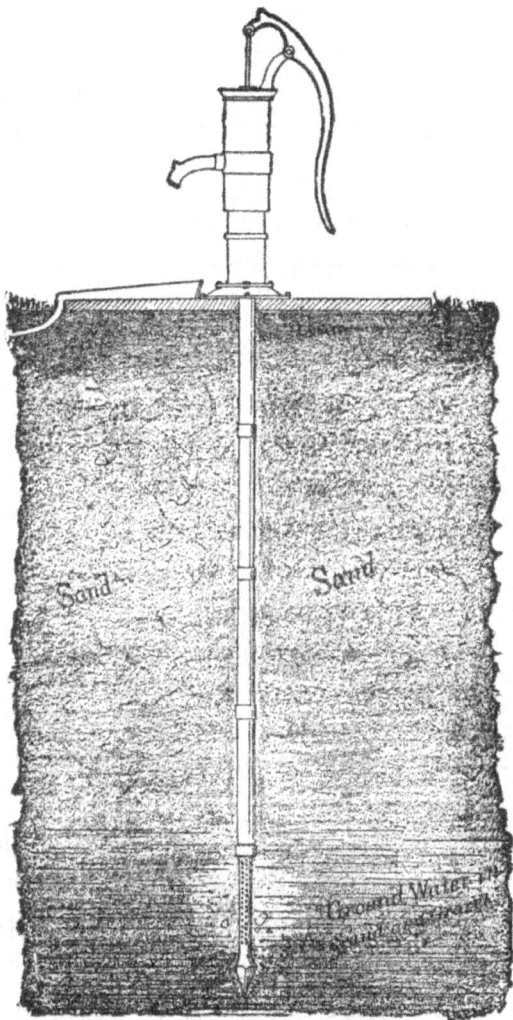

FIG. 3.—A DRIVEN WELL.

Now the purity of the water derived in all of these forms of wells from the ground water depends, so far as external contaminations are concerned, upon several things.

In the first place, the water which trickles down through the soil from the surface must not be so extraordinarily dirty, or in such large quantity, and the cleansing layers of soil must not be so thin that the water will not be well purified by natural filtration by the time it reaches the ground-water reservoirs. If in the case of an individual well, either dug or driven, the cesspools and the outhouses and the barns are situated so near the zone of soil drained by the well, that a proper filtration of the variously polluted water cannot occur, then the well water cannot be expected to be wholesome.

In the second place, while the ground-water supply coming in to the well at or near its bottom may be good and pure, it very often happens, especially in the old-fashioned dug and stoned wells, that channels of communication are in the course of time established between the contaminated surfaces of the ground about the well and the well itself, so that instead of being filtered, as it should be, slowly through considerable layers of soil, the surface water runs in at the sides between the stones at the upper part of the well, or even runs over the top edges directly in.

We want water for domestic use, just for the purpose of soiling it in the various processes of cleaning. It thus often happens, especially in the country, that a good deal of this soiling of water occurs very near the well, because in this way laborious carrying of the water is avoided. The soiled water is then either poured on to the ground close to the mouth of the well, or is carried but a short distance away to be emptied. The consequence of this is that the dirty water either runs in part directly back into the well again, or the soil for many feet about the well becomes gradually permeated with filth and no longer disposes, as it should, of the impurities soaking down towards the ground water, or more directly towards the well, after rains or after **the deluging of the surface with fresh dirty water.**

Finally, the open wells with a curb and a bucket, oaken or moss-covered though it be, permit a good deal of contamination of the well water from settling dust and from all sorts and conditions of things accidentally falling into it, or from the handling of the bucket with dirty hands. The coolness of the well, furthermore, often leads to its use as a refrigerator. Various kinds of food are lowered down towards the water, and not infrequently organic materials are spilled into it, which tend to make it a good culture medium for germs.

These considerations lead to a few precautionary sentences, which I shall ask the printer to emphasize.

Wells should not be dug in or near places where there is an unusual contamination of the soil with human or animal waste.

The surface of the ground for a few feet about the top of the well should be raised some inches above the general level; should slope away from the edge of the well, and be covered with water-tight cement or with bricks or stones cemented together, so that water from the surface cannot pass directly into the well at or near its mouth. There should be a separate drain to carry off the waste water.

The lining of the well, either brick or stone, should be cemented water-tight on all sides from the top to the bottom, so that all the water which enters may have passed through considerable thicknesses of soil.

The mouth of the well should be covered, to prevent foreign contaminating substances falling into the water, and for this reason, when it is practicable, it is better to use a pump than a bucket for drawing the water.

Finally, anybody found emptying dirty water or other foul material on to the surface or into pits in the soil near the well should—be he male or female—be subject to such domestic discipline or temporary disgrace as will call attention to the heinousness of his offence.

Fig. 4, which is copied from a drawing by Hueppe, shows the proper construction and surroundings of an ordinary shallow well. To indicate that either material may be used, the well is represented as bricked on one side and stoned on the other.   As the flat stone cover-

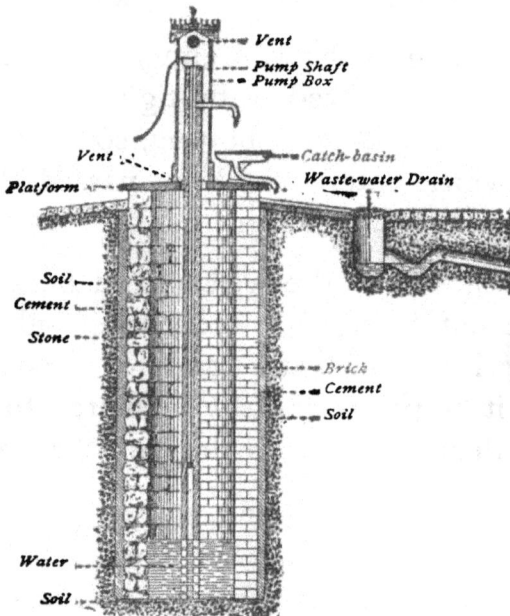

FIG. 4.—SKETCH OF A MODEL WELL.

ing the top is tightly cemented to the stone-or brick-work of the well and sealed tightly to the pump-house, a vent is made around the pump-shaft and another at the top, **covered** with a fine wire netting. It will be seen that in this well all the water must enter from the bottom, and will under all circumstances be secure from contaminations coming in from the immediate vicinity of the well.

The writer is conscious that just about here some disgusted householder is ready to pounce upon him, upbraiding him for destroying his peace of mind, and demanding why, then, in the name of all the worshippers at Hygeia's shrine, have not we well-water drinkers died off long ago ? What can we do with the household waste, if we must not hide it out of sight in the purlieus of our dooryards ? How far must the barnyards and cesspools and vaults be from the well to ensure for them the sanction of these new impertinent sanitary crusaders ?

In the calm which we hope will usher in the next chapter we will consider together some facts which bear upon these irate queries, and then endeavor to quell the perturbed spirit which we imagine to have just spoken here.

CHAPTER XII.

SOME LOOSE ENDS GATHERED UP.

WE have already seen that, so far as we yet know, it is but a very few of the bacteria which can cause harm to man. When we look over the known disease-producing forms, we find that it is but a small proportion even of these which are especially liable to be present in water.

We will now leave out of the account those forms of germs which, though ordinarily harmless, may, when present in large numbers, cause health disturbances in sensitive or very young persons, because we don't yet know very much about them and their life history. We will leave out of the account, too, those forms of disease-producing germs, which, as we conjecture but cannot yet prove, occasionally cause harm by getting into drinking-water,

—such as the germs of diphtheria and blood-poisoning and malaria.

When, now we take account of stock, we find that we have left two species of germs which we not only know can cause disease, but which have been repeatedly detected in polluted drinking-water. These are the bacteria of Asiatic cholera and of typhoid fever.

Thanks to the discovery of the germ of Asiatic cholera by Dr. Robert Koch, and the preventive measures which have been based upon our knowledge of its life history, the chances are slight that the reader of this page will ever be exposed to serious danger from its ravages, so that we may dismiss that germ too, with the single remark that the precautions which we must take to ward off the typhoid fever germ from our water supplies are equally applicable to the cholera germ.

Now at last we have at bay the actual enemy, which in the present stage of science seems the most formidable in connection with the pollution of water, namely, the Bacillus typhosus,—the cause and the only cause of typhoid fever. Let us look at this fellow, so prominent a figure in our bacterial rogues' gallery, for in him this cyclone of water sanitation is largely centred.

It is a short rather plump bacillus, very agile when swimming free in fluids, capable of rapid multiplication when under favorable conditions, and hardy too, unfortunately, so that it survives many serious vicissitudes of heat and cold, of drought and flood, with comparative nonchalance. It thrives under artificial cultivation in the laboratory, and, so far as we know, is found nowhere in nature except in the bodies of persons ill with typhoid fever, or in the waste material from such persons, which may get on to articles of food or into water. The typhoid bacillus can remain alive for a good while, and even for a time may multiply, in pure water. But after a while it dies off, unless it have more appropriate food than ordinary water furnishes. On the whole, it does not get along well in mixture with other and putrefactive germs. As we shall see later, it can resist considerable degrees of cold.

Such is the portrait and pedigree of the typhoid bacillus. The way in which it induces disease when it gets into the bodies of men we need not consider now. It should, however, be said that we do not know how many of the individual germs are necessary to set up the disease, nor do we know those conditions of the body which seem to predispose it to the incursions of the germs when once they do find a lodgment in it. We believe that these conservative powers of the body, which enable it to combat various deleterious agencies, are at some times more effective than at others. But this is a field yet to be explored.

The constancy of the supply of water from a well is, of course, dependent upon the extent and permanence of the ground-water supply of the region. Some wells penetrate the soil in a locality where the ground water is always present in abundance. Others are dependent, not upon a permanent accumulation, but upon an underground stream slowly working its way through the soil to a lower level. Such wells as the latter may be simply deep-lying cisterns, which catch the ground water flowing over them, and dry up when this ceases. Such a

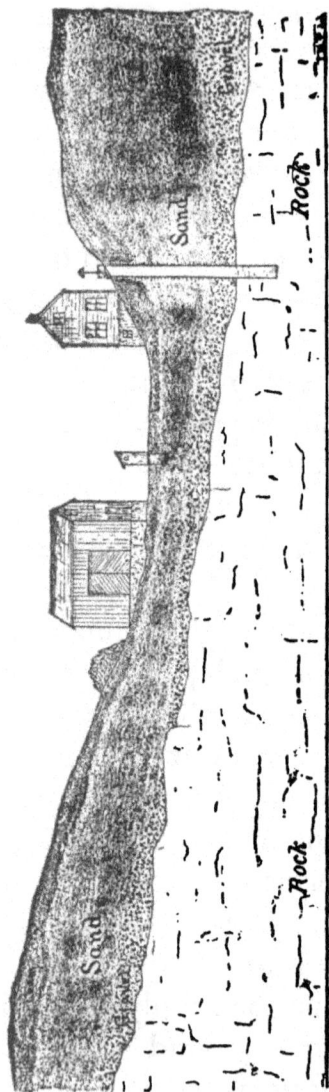

FIG. 5.—A CONTAMINATED WELL WITH INTERMITTENT SUPPLY FROM THE GROUND WATER.

94

well is shown in Fig. 5. The ground water here does not form a collection, but is slowly flowing along the rock surface from left to right through the gravel, and a portion of it is caught in the pit dug in the rock at the bottom of the well. This picture shows also that the situation of the well-curb at a higher level than the near sources of contamination of the water does not necessarily indicate that the well water is pure.

It will thus be seen that the direction of flow of the ground water is an extremely important matter for consideration when one is locating a well in regions not far removed from abundant soil contaminations.

We now come to the explanation of the presence among the living of our irate friend of the last chapter, who, as we suspect, felt guilty of the crime of permitting well and sewer contiguity, and attempted a game of bluff in demanding why in all reason, if we spoke the truth about wells, he was alive, he whose fathers and grandfathers as well as himself had always drunk water from open wells and out of the bucket too, and thrown the house waste just where they chose.

We are disposed to say to him for answer, venerable friend—there are indications in his tone that he may be getting on in years— venerable friend, if your cesspool and your barnyard and your necessary out-buildings are so near your well that the fluids from them may pass into the well without adequate natural filtration, or can pass unpurified into the ground-water reservoir which supplies your well ; or if you allow waste and dirty water to be thrown away near the opening of your well without a proper construction of the well's lining and top, you would be a great deal better occupied than in asking such questions, if you were down on your knees, returning thanks to an overruling Providence, which may have ordered it that among all the myriads of filthy and filth-breeding germs which have been swarming in your well perhaps for years, none of those particular forms have come which cause typhoid fever. Or, if the powers which rule over the destinies even of unsanitary people have not thought you worth that pro-

tection, it may be that your inherited robust-
ness, or your acquired vigor, or your love for
cider or some other beverage than water, may
have protected you from ill, even though the
danger germs have found their way to that
pit full of ground and sewer water, which you
call your well. Some of these, I think, are
the reasons why you are alive, and it is to be
hoped that you are alive enough to reform.

What shall you do with the waste stuff from
the household? Collect it in cans and sit up
nights to burn it, if you can't do any better.
Have it carted off frequently on to your land
far enough from the house to secure decent
cleanliness, at least. Or, if you have n't any
land outside your city lot, or small dooryard,
hire somebody to cart it off on to his. Use
earth closets, if you must. Run the kitchen
waste water far away from the well. Study
the soil and the rocks a bit in your region.
But don't stand on a compost heap near the
well-curb, and scream scorn and defiance at
anybody who comes along, and, for your own
good, tells you that no matter who makes
your clothes, no matter how much your house

7

costs, or how much you spend in scrubbings and Platt's Chlorides, you are essentially a dirty as well as a dangerous fellow, and ought to have been poisoned off before this, if you have n't.

The writer does n't propose to state just how many feet from the well the barnyard or the drain outlet may safely be, because these are questions which can only be answered one by one for each particular case. It is that the householder who is the arbiter of his own destinies in the matter of wells may be able to judge somewhat for himself of the necessities of the case, that we have gone so considerably into other domains to gather the foundations for an individual judgment.

Take the facts which may be gleaned from any good book on Hygiene, with some of the points in the new bacterial lore here so briefly set forth ; add to these an abundance of personal observation, and mix all with brains, and it will be a tough problem in water purveying which can't be solved without recourse to the analyst.

Ordinarily wells in populous towns or wherever they are near to out-buildings, drains, etc., are always liable to contamination, and should always be regarded with suspicion.

It should be distinctly understood by everybody that clearness and lack of bad taste in a water do not at all signify that it is free from dangerous impurity. Many millions of germs, harmful and harmless, may be present in a glass of water without in the slightest degree impairing its transparency to the naked eye.

While it has been many times proven that typhoid fever has been acquired by drinking water from wells polluted with sewage containing this germ, there is little doubt that, on the whole, polluted well water has been much too often assumed to have given rise to this contagion, without adequate proof. People are not sufficiently aware how readily the germ of typhoid may be carried from the sick to the well, in milk, on the surfaces of fruits and other articles of food, on the hands of attendants, and by flies which have had access to the undisinfected excreta.

There seems to be little to add here to what

has already been said in regard to the necessity for care and intelligence in the construction of wells, and in deciding upon their situation in reference to the depositing places of household waste. In fact, the marvellous cleansing powers of the soil may, when reasonable care has been exercised, be relied upon to prevent well-pollution under most ordinary conditions.

The wholesale and indiscriminate condemnation of wells, which one so frequently hears nowadays, as sources of family water supply, does not appear to be just. But so frequent are the offences against sanitary laws in the situation and construction of wells, that there is little doubt that it would be a positive benefit if at least half of the wells in the United States were to be closed forthwith.

CHAPTER XIII.

ARTIFICIAL WATER PURIFICATION.

WE have seen that Nature provides in a most efficient and liberal way for the purification of water on a large scale. We have seen that the difficulties in the way of getting pure water, either for large towns or for individual households, are largely due to the reprehensible way in which people allow their household or manufacturing waste to run into the natural sources of water supply, be they rivers, lakes, springs, or wells. We have learned that the most important polluting materials are those which come from the bodies of persons suffering from bacterial disease, because these materials are apt to contain living germs capable of inducing the same diseases in predisposed persons, when taken in with drinking-water.

We thus see that when we go back to the original sources of the trouble, we find that if the materials discharged from the bodies of the victims of bacterial diseases, and especially of typhoid fever and Asiatic cholera, were at once burned or received into disinfecting solutions of sufficient strength and allowed to remain there for a few hours, or until all the germs were killed, we should have taken the first great step towards the removal of the dangers of polluted water. Until this is done by the joint efforts of an intelligent people and conscientious physicians, reinforced by proper regulations established by the health authorities, all other efforts towards securing pure water in populous regions will be but inefficient makeshifts.

The second thing to be attended to is to secure such legislation as will as fully as possible prevent the access of sewage or other unhealthy waste to the sources of water supply, be they lakes or streams or wells. Such outrageous pollution of water used for drinking as goes on in the Hudson at and above Albany, or in the Schuylkill, from which Philadelphia is largely supplied, and in many other places in the land, is nothing short of criminal, and should be made legally so without delay.

The problem of sewage disposal is a very complex one, and needs more such careful study as has been going on for some time under the auspices of the Massachusetts Board of Health. But enough is already known about it to render wholly unjustifiable the present filthy practices which are permitted all over this land. The older countries have seen the folly of such wholesale poisoning of water sources, and have taken steps to prevent it.

It is a great pity that people are not more generally informed regarding some of the most excellent forms of cremating furnaces, in which all the garbage and all other waste from single households and public institutions, or from whole villages and even large cities, can be cheaply and easily destroyed. If this were done the whole problem of pure water supplies and of general cleanliness in both villages and cities would be brought a long way nearer to a favorable solution.

The prevention of water pollution is urgently demanded, not only in those water supplies which are already bad; but should be looked to in anticipation of the future in those supplies which are still fairly pure, but which are liable to become less and less so as the country around them becomes more populous. The Croton water supply of the great city of New York is in many respects an ideal one, and the Croton water is usually very good water indeed. But, before all other things connected with it—before new acqueducts, new distributing sources, new dams, new reservoirs, before all else—this one thing should be looked to, that the shores of the streams and lakes which furnish the water shall be absolutely protected from the entrance of human or animal or manufacturing waste.

Intelligent and stringent legislation is needed in this matter, or we shall wake some day to find our water polluted at its sources by the new habitations which are sure to cluster about them in the series of charming and attractive valleys where they lie.

We should not permit our attention to be

diverted from this absolute necessity by any loose talk about the colossal dilution which sewage would undergo if allowed to enter the Croton supplies, or about the long distances which it has to run, or about the self-purification which it may undergo on the way. All these favoring factors we should be glad of and cherish, but to prevent pollution at all hazards is the first thing.

He who is curious to learn just what entering wedges towards a pollution of our excellent Croton water may even now be observed, can consult the Report of the State Board of Health of New York, for the year 1889, in which will be found some pictorial intimations, more suggestive than savory of what we have to guard against.

One of these illustrations is reproduced in Fig. 6 (page 107).

Now, although there may be no direct pouring of sewage from these houses into this tributary to the Croton stream shown in the picture, a great variety of surface contaminations are liable to be washed into it during heavy rains. These contaminations may be ordinarily simply filthy. But let typhoid fever gain a foot-hold in the settlement and the stream might become dangerous as well as dirty.

The difficulty with the Croton water supply then, is not that it is always, or usually, or that it has ever been bad, but that it is liable at any time, temporarily at least, to become so, if the shores of the streams and reservoirs are not more carefully attended to.

The condition of the Croton water supply is typical of the supplies of many towns in this country, which, naturally excellent, are in danger of becoming bad and dangerous, as population increases, through lack of stringent legislation and intelligent and faithful inspection.

It will no doubt be always practically impossible to preserve absolutely pure the water supplies which originate, or are stored in, or which pass in open channels through populous regions. Under these conditions, it is now in many cases necessary, and with increasing frequency will become so, to subject the water to filtration or other forms of purification on the large scale.

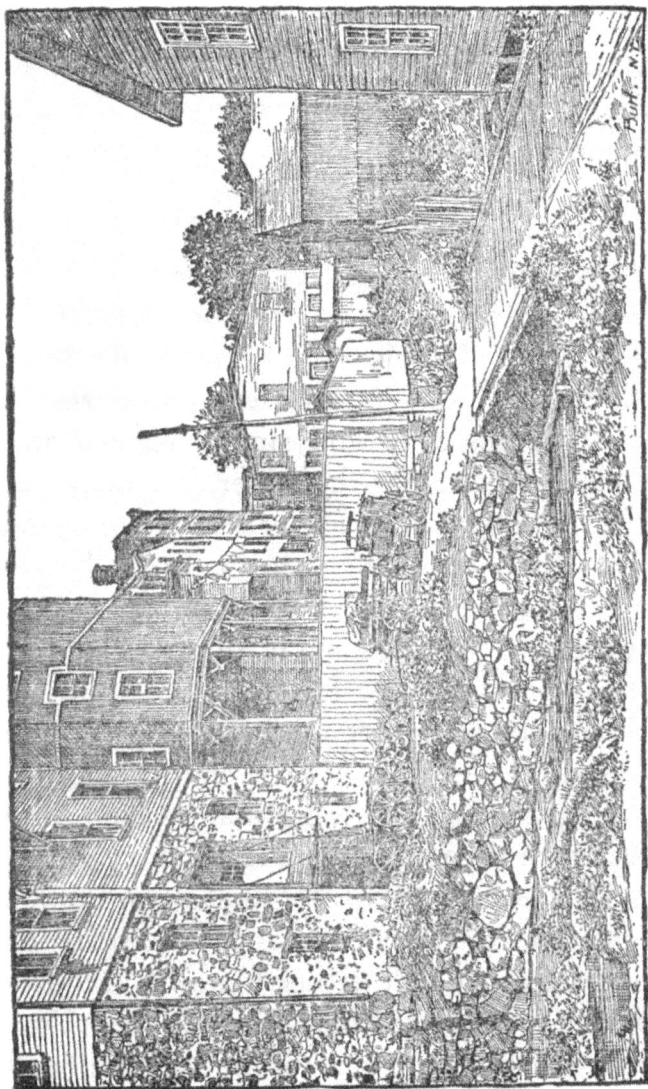

FIG. 6.—ONE OF THE TRIBUTARIES TO THE CROTON STREAM, SHOWING SOURCES OF CONTAMINATION OF THE WATER FROM ITS BANKS.

On the whole, the most successful proced-
ures in the way of artificial purification of water
for domestic use on the large scale have been
those in which Nature's modes of wholesale
soil filtration have been most closely imitated.
For this purpose, great filter beds are constructed, having stones at the bottom, and on
these layers of pebbles and gravel with sand
on the top. Now, it has been found that a
filter bed in this condition simply strains and
in a measure clarifies the water, but does not
remove its bacteria or its dissolved organic
matter. It is only when the layer of bacterial slime has been formed at the top, in the
way which we have studied in another chapter,
that the water may be largely freed from its
germs and its other organic pollutions. The
sand and gravel and stones simply afford a
supporting medium for the actual purifier—the
bacteria-formed pellicles and the hungry germs
which they enclose. Under these conditions,
however, the filtration must go on slowly or
the protecting pellicle either tears or becomes
inefficient, owing to the shortness of time
during which the water is in contact with
the cleansing layers.

While this in general is the way in which water is purified by the use of large filter beds, it has been found that if Nature be a little more closely imitated still, the results are better. In natural filtration in the soil the water does not lie, as a rule, very long at a time over the surface of the ground, but when the rain ceases, and the water soaks downward towards the ground-water reservoirs, the pores of the soil become more or less filled with air. Now the oxygen of the ground air seems to be a very necessary thing for the bacteria which tear polluting organic compounds to pieces in the process of natural filtration. So the intermittent character of the soil filtration has been copied in some artificial filter beds, which are not kept ceaselessly at work with their pores always full of water, but this is allowed frequently to settle through, so that the air may get into them when the surface is again flooded. Now the bacteria, in the presence of this new supply of oxygen, can tear apart and destroy much more completely than they could without it the polluting organic matter, should there be any such in the water.

There are many other modes of so-called

filtration and of water purification on the large scale. But this use of large filter beds in close imitation of Nature seems to be the most perfect of all the practicable cleansing processes now in use.

I do not say that some of the more rapid modes of water filtration on the large scale, such as are considerably used in this country, are not of value; but only that they have not, so far as I am aware, successfully sustained such practical and accurate tests as have shown the filter beds here described to be most efficient.

There are ways of removing foreign material from water by the addition of small quantities of chemicals which cause a voluminous precipitate, and these, on settling, may carry down a large part of the undesirable impurities. These precipitation methods are usually combined with some mode of filtration, and are regarded by many as very efficient. But as they are commonly applied to the purification of waters on the large scale, we need not dwell here upon their merits and demerits.

We have now finished with the large water supplies, their pollutions, and the means to prevent or partially to counteract them. These matters are mostly in the hands of experts, who should do for us on the large scale what the householder in the country must do for himself.

But, some one will say, what is the city householder to do, who either suspects or knows that the city water is not wholesome, in spite of the experts? Such things have been heard of as municipal governments which were much more concerned in gathering spoils for their administrators than in furnishing pure water and clean surroundings for the people.

The case is indeed a hard one, and the more difficult to treat from a scientific standpoint, because the professional politician is apparently one of those monstrosities who is not in accord either with nature or science or common-sense, and does n't fit into any system of reasonable living.

The remedy rests obviously enough with the citizens themselves, and it may be possible that some day respectable voters will realize in what serious jeopardy they place both health and life by the election of men to important municipal offices for their political affiliations and not for their fitness.

One, of course, thinks first, when confronted with the case of the town householder whose water supply is bad, of the small domestic filters. These, the writer is fully convinced, are, as a rule, a great deal worse than nothing. Almost all of them afford breeding-places for germs, and furnish water much richer in them after than before filtration. Most of them strain the water, and by thus removing some of the cruder, but for the most part harmless, impurities, make it look clearer and more attractive, but that, as a rule, is all.

There are one or two forms of small domestic filters which, if allowed to act very slowly, may remove a considerable proportion of the bacteria which polluted water contains. But all of the domestic filters which act rapidly are inefficient so far as the removal of bacteria is concerned. That this must be so is evident when we reflect upon the exceeding minuteness of these germs, which pass readily through pores large enough to permit the passage of large amount of water in a short time, especially under heavy pressure. Certain of the unglazed porcelain filters, such as the "Pasteur" and the "Berkefeldt," are the most reliable for household use ; but these must be frequently cleaned, and sterilized with great care, if fairly germ-free water is to be secured.

The small sand and sponge and cotton filters and others of their ilk, which screw on to the water faucet, and let large volumes of water rapidly through them, should be forthwith and definitely discarded, unless it be understood that they are simply strainers and not filters, and that their filling of whatever kind must be renewed every day.

In fact, the unhappy citizen who is supplied with dirty and dangerous water, will usually find his best security in boiling that portion which is to be used for drinking, as a matter of household routine, for half an hour. Or, if he can afford it, he may purchase for such use water which has been purified by distillation by some reliable manufacturer.

But these are all melancholy makeshifts, and should be looked upon solely as temporary devices to be employed only until the general

8

supply has been made wholesome. This can always be done, if only the people demand it with intelligent and unwearied insistance.

Enough has been said about wells and springs from which in general the rural house-holder gets his domestic supplies. It has been the aim of the writer in these chapters, not so much to lay down positive rules, which are often impracticable, as to place the reader on the vantage-ground of an intelligent student, who can deal with individual cases as they arise.

It will sometimes happen, though not nearly as often as might be imagined, that the aid of the chemist and bacteriologist must be summoned to pass judgment on a suspected source of water supply. When this is necessary, the analyst should be consulted as to the methods of collecting the water samples, and he should be as fully as possible informed about the surrounding and general condition of the source. It does not seem necessary here to describe the details of either chemical or biological analyses of water. The principles of the latter have been already set forth in the preceding books of this little series.

But it should be clearly understood by all who seek expert council in the matter of the salubrity of a given source of water supply, that it is seldom that the expert can definitely decide, either by a chemical or a biological analysis alone of a water sample, or by both together, the whole question of the purity and safety of the supply.

Very often, in fact usually, a far more positive and reliable opinion may be formed by an examination of the source itself and its surroundings than by an analysis, however searching, of a sample of the water. The examination of both the source and the water itself will usually lead the expert to a more useful opinion than if reliance be placed upon either method alone. The greatest usefulness of bacterial water analysis to-day depends upon its accuracy as a test of the efficiency of the filtration process to which water has been subjected. The seeker after more knowledge on the subject of water supplies may profitably consult the excellent work of Mason.

CHAPTER XIV.

SOLID WATER.

WE have thus far been studying water only in its liquid form. We may not forget, however, that in its gaseous condition as steam, water does a large part of man's heavy work in the world for him, and in the form of cloud-vapor does much to gratify his love of the beautiful. But water, in its solid form as ice, has in modern times become a very important factor in the physical well-being of man. In the United States not far from twenty-five millions of tons are annually cut and stowed away for the year's consumption.

The Hudson River has hitherto been the great source of ice supply for the city of New York, and some facts about the way in which it is gathered here may not be uninteresting, since it is fairly typical of the ice harvesting on the large scale all over the country.[1]

It is said that if all the ice-houses on the Hudson River below Albany were placed side by side, the line would be not far from seven miles long.

The better ice-houses, mostly of wood, have efficient drainage at the bottom. The walls are hollow, containing an air chamber, and within this a chamber filled with some non-conducting material, such as sawdust or hay, while above is a loft with abundant ventilation. The larger houses are divided into a number of rooms, so that when they are opened for the removal of the ice the whole mass need not be exposed to the warm air which enters.

The cakes of ice, which in this region are cut of a uniform size of about twenty-two by thirty-two inches, are usually laid flat, a solid stratum at the bottom. Above this they are placed on top of one another with two or three inches of space between their edges, the joints

[1] Through the courtesy of the publishers of that journal, the writer has been permitted to use in this and the following chapter some extracts from an article on ice, written by him some time ago for the *Popular Science Monthly.*

being broken every few tiers, as in masonry, by allowing the cakes to lap over the joints below. The object of the space between the edges of the cakes is to prevent their freezing together, for if this occurred their removal would entail a good deal of additional labor in breaking them apart, and a large loss of ice which would be chipped off in the operation. When the houses are about full, a solid layer of cakes is laid on top, so that the air may not circulate between them, and the whole is covered with hay. A varying number of smaller buildings are usually clustered about the storage-houses, such as engine-house, tool-house, shop, barn, and often the boarding-house for the men.

But let us leave these dry details and get out-of-doors, lest Winter should steal a march on us, and we should lose those first delicate crystal spiculæ shooting out from shore and rock with which he commonly begins his work alike on lake and stream and pool. Who does not know those fragile ice-fringes, losing themselves in the open water, which the first frosty nights in autumn leave behind often only to fade away in the next day's sun ? But when at length, after these early, playful exhibitions of his gathering power, Winter really bends himself to his work, the crystals grow longer and thicker, their sides join, and finally the completed film formed along the surface shuts in the water, and his dominion is complete. Now his tactics change. The caprices which he has displayed as the long crystals stole out in ever-varying directions from the shore are subdued, and the stern work of strengthening his fetters fairly begins.

After the first film of ice is formed, the freezing goes on directly downward as the heat from the water radiates off into the colder air above. The direction of crystallization has changed, and is now at right angles to that in which it began. Unhindered radiation of heat from the water out into the air is the secret of the continued formation of ice. If any thing occurs to prevent this, the ice stops forming beneath. A fall of snow upon the already made ice greatly retards its continued formation.

Some of the elder ice-harvesters still foster a feeble flame upon the broken altars of the old star-worshippers, in their belief that the cold rays from the winter moon and stars favor in some mysterious way the growth of their ice, since this forms best on clearest nights. Who would dispel this chaste illusion by suggesting that the clouds which draw themselves at times over the faces of their gentle deities delay the fruition of their hopes simply by preventing the escape of the earth's heat off into space?

In the vicinity of New York, where open winters are so common and changes of temperature are so great and frequent, the formation of the ice is a matter of the greatest solicitude to the ice-farmer, upon whose vigilance and judgment may largely depend both the value and abundance of his winter's crop.

While the weather is clear and cold, and the colder and clearer the better, all goes well with the growing crop, as slowly the water yields itself into its crystal bonds, and the domain of the clear solid ice creeps downward inch by inch. But this condition of affairs, quite ideal from the standpoint of the ice-farmer, is apt in this region to be evanescent. If the grip of the cold relaxes by day, the formation of ice may stop, and even a film of that already made may melt away in the water beneath ; but at night again another layer may be added, and so, with many halts, retreats, and slow advances, little by little the ice-mass thickens. But who would imagine that, written in the ice, as plainly as the sequence of geologic ages is written in the rocks, is the record of these alternate victories of heat and cold, as they contended for the mastery of the water during the winter days and nights? Strange as it may seem, the record is there, however, and, stranger yet, is written in air.

Look at the edge of a cake of ice which has formed in comparatively still water during such alternations of temperature as are common in our winters, and you will be very apt to see a series of bands of transparent ice, between which lie layers of tiny air bubbles. In still water, when the ice for any reason stops forming for a time, bubbles of air from the water or from the bottom are apt to rise and collect beneath the ice, and when the freezing again begins they are entangled and held fast between the old and the new ice-layers, a permanent record of the relaxation of the thrall of the cold long enough for their collection. In running water such bubbles are apt to be swept away, and the ice remains transparent.

While the ice is thus forming the ice-farmer looks on, his spirits rising in inverse ratio to the height of the thermometer. To the vagaries of the temperature he must reconcile himself as best he may. But let his *bête noire*, the snow—if so violent an antithesis be permissible—appear, and he will be on the alert at once. The snow-flakes, delicately adjusting themselves to one another as they settle down upon the ice, build up among their crystals myriads of tiny air cavities, and the whole forms a veritable blanket which hinders radiation. It is warm for the same reason that a down comfortable is—it prevents the escape of heat. Now, what shall our ice-farmer do? It does little good to swear at the snow, although he usually has recourse to this procedure first. If the already formed ice is thick enough to bear the teams, he may scrape the snow off, and then the freezing can go on. But if not, he sends his men over the field to cut small holes here and there through it ; the water wells up, flows over the top, forming a layer of slush, a good deal of the air is expelled, and the whole freezes, forming a whitish layer which is called snow ice.

This layer is whitish because of the air bubbles which it still retains, but it conducts off the heat fairly well, and his crop goes on forming. This operation is called "tapping" or "bleeding" the ice. Ice which has a very thick snow layer is called "fat ice." This snow ice is not as valuable as clear ice, for householders object to it because they fancy that it is not so pure, and the assurances of the dealers that the impurity is only air appear to have little weight. So the more responsible dealers usually find it for their interest to remove most of the snow layer. A little snow ice on the cakes, however, makes them keep better. We shall see by and by that there are really very good reasons why the snow ice from certain sources should not be used for drinking purposes.

Too much ice must not be grooved out by the ploughs in advance, lest in case of rain the channels should fill and freeze solid, and the labor be wasted. So it is frequently necessary for the workers at the plough to be out long before light in the morning, grooving out blocks for the harvesters when the day begins. It is a picturesque sight—these hardy men, muffled to their ears, following the gingerly treading teams back and forth over the ice-fields by the light of flaring, smoky torches, hung on poles stuck in the ice. More than once the swinging lamps, which have done patriotic duty in some campaign torch-light procession, have found themselves relegated to the austere and chilling duty of illuminating hoary ice-fields before the dawn, instead of lending force to the political claims and convictions of would-be or would-continue-to-be American statesmen after dark.

At last the vicissitudes and anxieties of the growth of the ice crop are over, and the "boss" decides that the cutting shall begin. The first step in the ice gathering is to draw two long, straight lines on the ice at right angles to each other. With these as a guide, a part of the field is marked off into blocks of the proper size, and it then looks like a gigantic checker-board. Then other teams come on, drawing the ice-ploughs, which are long, narrow-toothed blades, running along the ice like great horizontal saws. One plough follows another along these narrow grooves until they are deep enough, so that long strips of the outlined cakes may be readily loosened by a saw. These separated strips of ice, grooved off into cakes, are pushed along in a channel which has been cleared through the ice up to the foot of the endless chain which runs up an incline to the houses. Here the strips are broken apart along the deep cross-grooves into cakes by hand-bars shaped like chisels.

The cakes are now caught upon projections from the elevating chain, moved by steam, and up they go, one after another, to the platforms at varying heights around the ice-houses, or directly in at the main door. When the cakes enter the storage-rooms they are shoved along wooden runs or movable tracks to various parts of the chamber, where, layer by layer, they are stowed away. Sometimes a single inclined plane with its endless chain leads up to a series of platforms along the front of the building, which tier above tier slope gently away from the top of the incline, so that the ice-cakes, leaving the chain at the centre, are slid down the platforms to the various openings.

The ice mass, which is quite imposing as one looks across it in the larger houses, must be carefully and skilfully packed, and be self-supporting. Many a dealer has come to grief by the fall of his building from the collapse of the ice mass within. The construction of the great and elaborate ice palaces with which the people of Montreal and St. Paul sometimes amuse themselves in winter is comparatively simple, because water is poured in between the blocks, and the whole freezes to a solid mass as it rises. But the art of the commercial ice-builder consists in making his ice mass solid enough to stand alone, with just as little freezing together of the cakes as possible.

CHAPTER XV.

THERE is yet another phase in the story of the ice which we must not overlook. We have been wont to believe that the fragment of ice, which forms such a constant and pleasing adjunct to our glass of water, is the very ideal of purity. But the common belief that, in freezing, water purifies itself from all kinds of contamination, has been shown to be quite untrue; and, ungraceful as is the task of dispelling so pleasing an illusion, we shall do unwisely if we ignore the revelations of modern science, and for the sake of a momentary mental quietude remain oblivious to a real danger, which the indiscriminate use of ice for drinking purposes unquestionably entails.

He who is familiar with the researches of Tyndall and other physicists on the structure of ice, knows how little we can be aware, from the simple inspection of a lump of clear ice, beautiful as it is, how marvellously it is built up, crystal by crystal, into the solid form we know so well. But if we turn a beam of sunlight upon it, concentrated by a lens, the exquisite and varied stellate figures which flash out within the solid mass as the magic touch of the sunbeam releases the molecules of water from their crystal bonds give us enchanting glimpses of the still but half-won secrets of beauty and of order with which Nature so fondly sports and still so cleverly conceals.

But the resources of the physicists do not suffice to conjure all its secrets from a block of ice. It is left for the student of that phase of nature which we call life to discover that this very type of cold impassive lifelessness may be fairly teeming, absolutely transparent though it be, with whole families and races of living things—dormant from chill, it is true, but ready at the touch of warmth and in the presence of their food to start on a career of growth and multiplication, to which the increase in the world's populousness, since the old Ice age faded, is but a poor and halting comparison.

We cannot follow the student of these lowly forms of life, which have become entangled among the ice crystals, as he calls them back from their torpor, separates them one by one, and patiently studies their life history. It is not enough to melt the ice and look at the resulting water through the microscope. But he plants the melted ice in good bacterial food, and studies the forms which grow, and finds out how numerous they are.

A great deal of careful experiment has shown that water in freezing largely expels its coarser visible contaminations, and also that a large proportion of the invisible bacteria which it contains may be destroyed, even as many as ninety per cent. But still large numbers may remain alive, for many species are quite invulnerable to the action of cold. It has been found that in ice formed from water containing many bacteria, such as water with sewage contaminations, the snow-ice almost invariably contains many more living bacteria than the more solid, transparent part ; so that the snow-layer should be especially avoided in ice obtained from questionable sources.

Unfortunately the bacteria which cause typhoid fever are not readily killed by cold, and may remain alive for months, fast frozen in a block of ice. But the typhoid-fever germ can be present in water, so far as we know, only when it is contaminated with refuse from persons suffering from the disease ; so that, if we can be certain that our ice was cut from water uncontaminated with sewage or human waste, we have nothing to fear from its use so far as this disease is concerned.

A considerable part of the ice supplied in ordinary seasons to New York and Brooklyn is cut on the Hudson River, and much of it just below Albany, where the stream is so greatly contaminated with the sewage of two large towns, Troy and Albany, as to be absolutely filthy. In both of these towns typhoid fever is of frequent occurrence during the period in which ice is forming, and the waste from the victims passes directly into the river. There would, therefore, seem to be a very real danger in the use of some of the Hudson River ice.

The responses which one commonly meets when he has occasion to point out the possibility of danger from the use of impure ice are apt to be: "How horrid. Why do you add another misery to life?" or, "Our fathers have never suffered from the use of ice, and why should we?" etc. No sanitary danger has ever been pointed out, and no improvement instituted, which had not to stem just such opposition. The cesspool has given way to the sewer, and the town-well to the distant water supply, in the face of the same sort of silly protest on the part of many of those whose own most vital interests were at stake—persons who ignore the fact that an ever-increasing vigilance is necessary to ward off the dangers which the aggregation of large numbers of people in cities invariably entails.

The danger from the use of impure ice in New York, though widespread, is not very alarming, so far as the liability to extensive outbreaks of typhoid-fever are concerned, because most of the ice which is furnished appears to be of fair quality. But if the risk of an attack of the disease can be warded off from one in ten thousand of our fellows, the gain is worth the effort. We do not need to be unduly squeamish, but it is well enough to be intelligent in the face of sanitary dangers.

The ice companies, unless controlled by the State Health Department, will doubtless continue to cut and to furnish sewage ice along with the rest just as long as their customers will tolerate it. But if householders would insist upon the assurance that their ice should not come from the immediate vicinity of Albany, or from directly below other towns draining into the river, the companies would soon recognize that acquiescence in this reasonable demand is the wiser and more profitable course.

We have entered into the details of the New York ice supply because it illustrates conditions which are found everywhere in this country where natural ice is cut and stored for sale.

Ice-water is so cold that the nerves of taste are temporarily benumbed, and so the bad taste of much of the filthy ice goes unnoticed, and we are not warned, as we are in the use of some bad waters used at a more moderate temperature. Then again, it should not be forgotten that many millions of living germs may be present in a bit of ice no larger than a hen's egg, and yet its beautiful transparency may not be in the least degree impaired.

It may be regarded as a safe practical rule, that a body of water which from its conditions and surroundings would not be considered as a good source of water supply should not be used to cut ice from ; and this test is perhaps after all quite as valuable as are the more subtle methods of the analyst.

If the householder be not brave enough to encounter the scorn of the ice-dealer, or is too tender-hearted to witness the picture of injured innocence which he often presents when the details of his business are called in question, the ice which is used for drinking purposes may be put in a separate receptacle, so as not to come directly in contact with the water.

CHAPTER XVI.

ARTIFICIAL ICE.

OUR space does not permit us to consider the growing importance of the manufacture of artificial ice. But it seems probable that the sanitary problems which the use of natural ice for drinking purposes presents, especially in large cities, may find their solution in the increasing employment of artificial ice made from distilled or otherwise purified water, or from good natural water.

In regions where the sources of ice are good, and the consumer can ascertain what they actually are, the natural ice will most likely continue, as it should, to afford the general supply. But in cities like New York, whose supply comes so largely from a grossly polluted source, and where the householder has no security that the dealer will not furnish him with this polluted ice when the name of the company implies a supply from better sources, there should be little hesitation on the part of the consumer to use the artificial ice just as soon as it is furnished at reasonable rates, and the details of its manufacture are found to be cleanly.

There has been an attempt in some quarters to create and foster a prejudice against artificial ice because ammonia is used in the common process of manufacture. The writer has heard it gravely stated by the *attachés* of the natural-ice companies that the bubbles in artificial ice were caused by the ammonia which it contained; and in one instance ammonia was metamorphosed into "pneumonia," in the solemn warning. It seems hardly necessary to say here that the ammonia does not come in contact with the water which is frozen; and the bubbles which are frequently seen in cakes of artificial ice are no more due to chemicals used in its manufacture than are the bubbles frequently so abundant in natural ice.

In the cakes of artificial ice which are already becoming familiar in our streets, one usually sees a curious whiter central portion, made up of air bubbles, in the largely transparent block.

The water in the common process of ice manufacture is placed in large metallic cans of the shape and size of the finished ice-cake. These cans are surrounded by the cooling material, and the freezing commences at the sides of the can. The ice crystals shoot out at right angles to the cooling surfaces, just as they do in the formation of natural ice, and as they coalesce at their sides they squeeze out the air which the water contained in the form of bubbles, and crowd it along in front of them as freezing proceeds. One result of this is that when finally the ice walls advancing from all four sides of the cans towards the centre meet, the varying numbers of air bubbles entangled at the tips of the ice crystals are imprisoned at the centre, forming the whiter bubbly centre of the block.

Not infrequently, one sees in the artificial-ice blocks narrow bubbly streaks extending from the corners of the block to the central bubbly mass. These are formed in the same way, and indicate the line of meeting of the ice crystals, which shot out near the corners when the earliest parts of the ice were formed and met at right angles.

To see the methods of freezing and removing the blocks of artificial ice from the cans, and the devices for handling them, is well worth a visit to one of the artificial-ice manufactories.

CHAPTER XVII.

THE LAST WORD.

WE have seen in our hurried glances at water and its use by man, that good old Mother Nature has made ample provision for us, and that we need have little to fear from bad water, either in town or country, if only we pay due regard to her teachings, and look to it that our surroundings are kept clean.

Vast hordes of tiny toilers at her behest are working in our service day and night to keep the world wholesome, and all the races of beings supplied with life-stuff.

We have found an invisible flora in the water, and have learned that for the most part it bodes no ill to man. We have learned that we can nurse back to life the delicate organisms which were sporting in the water when it fell under the spell of Winter's wand, and wring from them, one by one, the secret of their human relationships.

It is certain that the wholesale curtailment of many forms of disease may be brought about by rigid attention to some of the simplest details of sanitation.

It has become plain that the new science of bacteriology has done much to make this prevention of disease possible. It is, however, equally plain that by unceasing and intelligent vigilance alone, on the part of all, can we achieve that end.

But do not be discouraged, patient reader, nor let the burden of modern cleanliness rest too heavily in your consciousness. The obvious necessities in this direction will be easily enough met when their fulfilment becomes habitual.

Our leaf-clad forefather no doubt protested with all the forcefulness of pristine expletives, as, day by day, he was reminded that the refuse of the little housekeeping must be deposited farther and farther from the tent. And clear down to our own day and hour, every suggestion of sanitary reform has encountered protest, and its promulgators have incurred the odium of soul-disquieting nuisances.

The standards of cleanly living rise, because the obstacles become greater, and the aim higher and more comprehensive. But little by little, cleanliness has won its way to favor, and man has always been the better for it in the end.

INDEX.

THE END.

HEALTH NOTES FOR STUDENTS. By
BURT G. WILDER, M.D., Professor of Physiology,
Cornell University and the Medical School of Maine.
Paper . . . . 20 cts

A SELECTION FROM THE CONTENTS.

Maxims and General Remarks ; Choice of Room ; Drainage ;
Food and Drink ; Ventilation and Heating ; Clothing ; Bathing ;
Care of the Hands, etc. ; Sleep—Its Importance to Students ;
Exercise ; Methods of Study ; Care of the Eyes ; Stimulants
and Narcotics ; Hygiene and Morality.

" They are admirable, and within the reach of everybody in
this highly condensed form."—*Post*, Hartford.

" It is full of practical and thoroughly sensible suggestions,
concisely and clearly phrased."—*Courier*, Boston.

" Its attentive perusal would prolong the life and preserve
the health of many a young man, be he student or no student."
—*Phila. Inquirer.*

" If this simple, brief advice could be mentally digested by
every one, the labors of the medical profession would be materially lightened."—*American.*

" Many thanks for the ' Health Notes ' which ought to be very
useful, as they will be, I trust, among our young men, who are
in great need of such advice, at all times, and everywhere."—
OLIVER WENDELL HOLMES, Nov. 8, 1883.

G. P. PUTNAM'S SONS,   NEW YORK.

www.ingramcontent.com/pod-product-compliance
Lightning Source LLC
Chambersburg PA
CBHW070929210326
41520CB00021B/6865